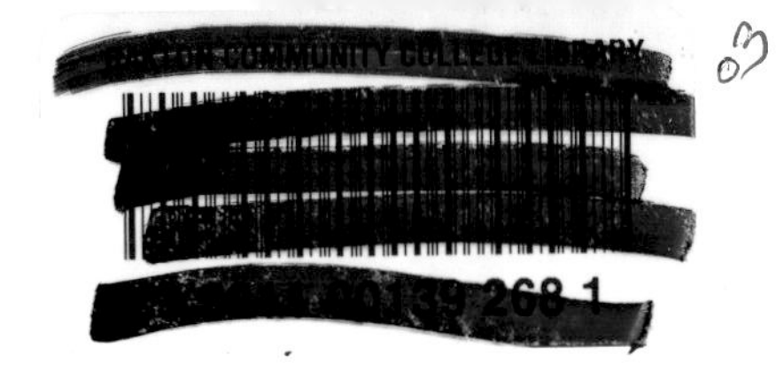

Sleep Disorders

Sleep Disorders: Diagnosis, Management and Treatment
A handbook for clinicians

Peretz Lavie, PhD
Andre Ballard Professor of Biological Psychiatry and
Head of Technion Sleep Laboratory,
Faculty of Medicine,
Technion – Israel Institute of Technology,
Haifa, Israel

Giora Pillar, PhD, MD
Physician, Sleep Laboratory, and Pediatrics Department
Rambam Medical Centre,
and Senior Lecturer,
Faculty of Medicine
Technion – Israel Institute of Technology,
Haifa, Israel

Atul Malhotra, MD
Specialist in Pulmonary and Critical Care,
Brigham and Women's Hospital and
Instructor, Harvard Medical School,
Boston, USA

MARTIN DUNITZ

First published in the United Kingdom in 2002
by Martin Dunitz Ltd, The Livery House, 7–9 Pratt Street, London NW1 0AE

Tel.: +44 (0) 20 7482 2202
Fax.: +44 (0) 20 7267 0159
E-mail: info@dunitz.co.uk
Website: http://www.dunitz.co.uk

A CIP record for this book is available from the British Library.

ISBN 1-84184-055-6

Distributed in the USA by
Fulfilment Center
Taylor & Francis
7625 Empire Drive
Florence, KY 41042, USA
Toll Free Tel: +1 800 634 7064
E-mail: cserve@routledge_ny.com

Distributed in Canada by
Taylor & Francis
74 Rolark Drive
Scarborough, Ontario M1R 4G2, Canada
Toll Free Tel: +1 877 226 2237
E-mail: tal_fran@istar.ca

Distributed in the rest of the world by
Thomson Publishing Services Ltd.
Cheriton House
North Way
Andover, Hampshire SP10 5BE, UK
Tel:+44 (0)1264 332424
E-mail: salesorder.tandf@thomsonpublishingservices.co.uk

The front cover design incorporates artwork by Grazia De Tommasi

Composition by Wearset Ltd, Boldon, Tyne and Wear

Printed and bound in Malta by The Gutenberg Press Ltd

Contents

Preface

Although sleep and dreams have attracted human interest since the dawn of history, it has only been in the last 30 years that physicians have recognized the importance of sleep disorders, and no more than 20 years since objective diagnostic procedures have been routinely employed for their diagnosis. With a growing number of sleep clinics and sleep laboratory evaluations, we are witnessing the emergence of the new field of sleep medicine. This rapidly growing field attracts physicians from diverse disciplines, such as pulmonology, internal medicine, psychiatry, neurology, otolaryngology, paediatrics, and even dentists, all of whom are now becoming 'sleep physicians' after appropriate training. Humans sleep between a quarter and a third of their lives, and many complain of sleep disturbances. The overall prevalence of sleep problems may be as high as 30% in children and adults, and even higher in elderly people. These sleep disorders are diverse, and in order to deal with all of them a systematic classification is required. Over the years, several classifications have been proposed for sleep disturbances, including those based on symptoms, the origin of the disturbance, objective measurements, etc. As this book aims to serve primarily primary care personnel who may need to deal with patients with sleep disorders, we chose to discuss sleep disorders chiefly based on symptoms.

Based on this approach, sleep disturbances can be classified into one of four groups: insomnias, hypersomnias, parasomnias and sleep–wake schedule disorders. Insomnia describes a condition when a patient is tired, desires to sleep, yet suffers from any combination of difficulties falling asleep, difficulties maintaining sleep and early morning awakening. Hypersomnia, on the other hand, describes a condition when patients remain sleepy, usually despite adequate sleep time. Parasomnias are undesired events occurring during sleep, and sleep–wake schedule disorders (known also as circadian rhythm abnormalities) reflect a situation in which patients sleep at undesired times. Since in most cases of sleep–wake disorders the presenting symptoms are suggestive of insomnia, we incorporated this group under insomnia. Intentionally, we placed a greater emphasis on the hypersomnias and in particular sleep apnoea syndrome. The reason is that the vast majority of patients who spend their nights in sleep laboratories around the world for clinical examination, do so because of complaints related to excessive daytime sleepiness, non-refreshing sleep and chronic fatigue that cannot be ameliorated by sleep, in 80–90% of them, laboratory examination uncovers breathing disorders in sleep.

Theoretically, symptom approach to sleep disorders could be an easy and logical classification; however, in reality it is complicated by a considerable amount of overlap between the different groups. Notably, sleep apnoea syndrome can be manifested as a disorder of excessive somnolence; it is not uncommon to encounter a sleep apnoea patient whose chief complaints are of initiating and maintaining sleep. Thus, whenever there is an overlap and specific diagnoses can result in several symptoms this is pointed out and discussed. The appendix provides a brief summary of the *International Classification of Sleep Disorders*, which was developed in a manner compatible with the widely used ICD (*International Classification of Diseases*) in medicine in general.

Based on this approach, historically, sleep disturbances were classified into one of two groups:

1 sleep disorders with no organic origin, ICD 307.4,
2 the sleep disturbances, ICD 780.5.

The ICSD therefore kept the same codes given in the ICD classification for specific diagnoses, and gave original codes for new diagnoses.

This book will be of interest to clinicians and sleep specialists, and also will be particularly appropriate for the non-specialist. It highlights the most important issues in sleep medicine that the general practitioner may be facing in his or her daily practice. It covers basic sleep physiology, pathophysiology of sleep disorders, effective treatment procedures and long-term management of all sleep disorders. It is written in a factual and systematic manner, examining the entire area of sleep and its disorders. Our goal is to provide an invaluable, much-needed reference guide for the clinician. The authors rely on their vast experience in this field in establishing diagnostic sleep centres and treatment programmes both in Israel and in the USA.

Peretz Lavie, Giora Pillar and Atul Malhotra
Haifa, Israel 2002

chapter 1

History of sleep medicine

Sleep and dreams have been popular throughout time for writers, researchers and physicians alike. However, most of our modern knowledge of sleep medicine was achieved only in the last four decades. There have been several breakthrough discoveries that paved the way to the scientific investigation of sleep (Table 1).

To date, the understanding of why we sleep and the precise sleep control mechanisms of the brain are far from being completely elucidated. Previously, it was believed that sleep is a time of quiescence and

Table 1 Hallmarks of sleep research

1907	Induction of sleep in non-sleepy dogs using serum of sleep-deprived dogs (Legendre and Pieron). Took the hypnotoxin theory to its zenith
1920	Sleep deprivation results in greater sleepiness in the night than the following morning (Kleitman). Increased the understanding of the circadian drive to sleep
1928	The discovery of the electroencephalogram (EEG, Hans Berger). Enabled the possibility of measuring sleep objectively
1949	Electrical stimulations of the brain. The discovery of the reticular formation (Moruzzi and Magoun)
1953	The discovery of rapid eye movement (REM) sleep (Aserinsky and Kleitman)

tranquillity, a time when the body and mind relax to recuperate from the day's activity, a time when relatively little happens. These assumptions are partially incorrect because sleep is, in fact, an active process. At the start of the nineteenth century, the major sleep theory was that of the hypnotoxins. This theory posited that when we are awake there is an accumulation of poisonous hypnotoxin which drives sleepiness. Hypnotoxins were thought to be detoxified only during sleep. The discovery that serum from sleep-deprived dogs injected into alert dogs caused them to fall asleep (Legendre and Pieron) provided strong support for this theory.

Currently, several mediators, such as adenosine, interleukins, tumour-necrosing factor, prostaglandins, lipopolysaccharides and δ-producing proteins, have been proposed to mediate the homoeostatic drive for sleep. Sleep, however, is not regulated by just homoeostatic principles. The discovery by Kleitman that, even with on-going sleep deprivation, one can be less sleepy the following morning suggested that additional factors control the drive for sleep. Indeed, the current agreement among sleep researchers is that sleep is regulated by two factors: the duration of wakefulness (homoeostatic drive to sleep) and the time of day (circadian drive to sleep). The absolute drive to sleep at any point in time is therefore the combination of these two drives.

The discovery of the electroencephalogram in 1928 by Berger provided a quantum leap for sleep research. Applying the new methods to

Table 2 Physiological characteristics of the various stages of sleep

	EEG	*EMG*	*EOG*
Wake	β, α	Very high	Rapid
Stage 1	Some θ	High	Slow
Stage 2	θ, spindles	Some	Rare
Stage 3	Moderate δ	Low	Rare
Stage 4	Much δ	Low	Rare
REM sleep	Fast (θ, α)	Absent	Rapid

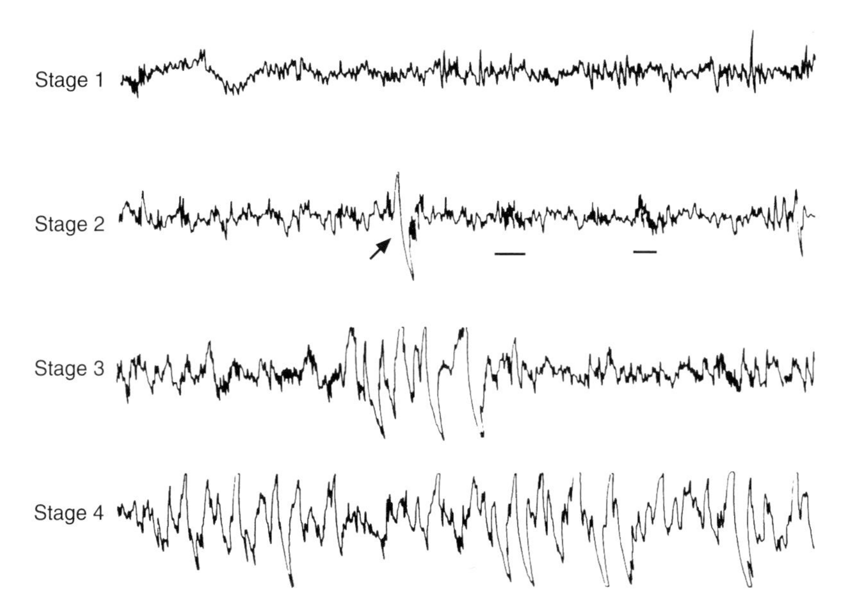

Figure 1 *EEG examples from the various sleep stages. (See text for further explanation.)*

measure EEG activity in sleeping people, or animals, revealed that the transition from wakefulness to sleep is accompanied by specific and well-characterized changes in brain wave activity (Table 2 and Figure 1). Electrocephalography (EEG) has allowed widespread investigations of brain mechanisms controlling sleep and wakefulness by several investgators, including Frederick Bremer, Moruzzi and Magoun, Michele Jouvet and others. There is still an on-going effort for further understanding of the brain circuitry participating in sleep regulation.

Normal sleep

During sleep there are periods of physiological and autonomic activation reaching waking levels. EEG and other physiological recordings during sleep define two distinct states of sleep: rapid eye movement (REM) sleep and non-REM (NREM) sleep. The latter is divided into four different stages: stage 1 (light sleep), stage 2 (consolidated sleep), and stages 3 and 4 (deep, or slow wave sleep). Division of sleep into these stages relies on three physiological variables: EEG, electromyography (EMG) and electro-oculography (EOG) as demonstrated in Table 2 and Figure 1.

The different EEG patterns that are characteristic of non-REM sleep stages are shown in Figure 1. Stage 1 is characterized by relatively low-amplitude θ activity intermixed with episodes of α activity. In stage 2 there are K-complexes (marked with an arrow) and sleep spindles (marked by underlining), whereas stages 3 and 4 are dominated by increasing amounts of slow-wave high-amplitude (δ) activity.

During normal sleep, these stages tend to occur in succession, forming a unique 'sleep architecture' (see Chapter 2). Generally, from wakefulness an individual falls into stage 1 sleep, followed by stages 2, 3 and 4 and REM sleep. This succession of sleep stages, culminating in REM sleep, forms a 'sleep cycle'. The length and content of sleep cycles change ...oughout the night as well as with age. The relative percentage of deep ...hest in the first sleep cycle and decreases as the night pro- ...ereas the relative length of REM sleep episodes increases ...t the course of the night. When totalling the various sleep ...ough the night in normal young adults, stage 1 occupies up to ... night, stage 2, 50%, and REM sleep and slow wave sleep (SWS) ... each. These relative percentages change with age, as does the ...gth. In infants the normal cycle of sleep lasts about an hour, ... in adults it lasts about 1.5 hours. Table 3 demonstrates the per- ...s of different sleep stages and sleep length at different ages.

... body movements, which may be accompanied by arousals, mark transitions to and from REM sleep. These four to eight brief awakenings, which are too short to be registered in the memory, are not considered abnormal or sleep disruption. This point is important to keep in mind when dealing with complaints about sleep. It is the difficulty in falling back to sleep, once brief awakening has occurred, rather than the awakenings themselves that may need to be treated. In some sleep disturbances, however, there is a large increase in the number of brief arousals from sleep, which indeed needs medical attention.

Table 3 Changes in sleep content and length with age

	Sleep time (h)	*Stages 1–2 (%)*	*Stages 3–4 (%)*	*REM (%)*
Infants	13–16	10–30	30–40	40–50
Children	8–12	40–60	20–30	20–30
Adults	6–9	45–60	15–25	15–25
Elderly people	5–8	50–80	5–15	15–25

Sleep needs and the function of sleep

One of the most popular questions that almost every sleep expert is faced with is 'How many hours do I need to sleep?'. As presented in Table 3, total hours of sleep are age dependent. Within each age group, however, there are large individual differences in sleep need. Of individuals in the general adult population, 97% sleep between 6 and 9 hours per day. When young adults were instructed to remain in bed for 16 hours in darkness per day for a 1-month period, their total sleep time stabilized at 8.5 h. This may represent the true sleep need. Sleeping less than 6 hours a night generally results in symptoms of sleep deprivation (see below). Interestingly, sleeping excessively may also result in non-refreshing sleep and daytime fatigue.

Thus, one cannot prepare a 'sleep bank' for future needs. There have been several well-publicized studies examining the limits of sleep needs, and whether these can be modified. In one such study, conducted by the US Navy, it was suggested that people who sleep regularly for 8 hours per night are able to reduce their sleep time gradually to 7 or 7.5 hours, without experiencing symptoms of sleep deprivation. This conclusion has, however, been refuted in most modern studies. It has been shown that even moderate sleep curtailment, when experienced for several days, impairs daytime alertness and performance. On the other hand, increasing sleep even from 7 to 8 hours improves quality of life as well as daytime cognitive functioning. Thus, total sleep time should be adequately assessed in the differential diagnosis of daytime sleepiness and chronic fatigue.

The first step in the approach to find out the causes of excessive sleepiness is to eliminate partial sleep deprivation as a possible cause. It should be remembered that, for some individuals, sleep need is as high as 9–10 hours a night, whereas they may sleep no more than 7 h per night. If sleepiness disappears after an adequate amount of sleep is achieved, as frequently happens at weekends, then sleepiness was most probably caused by partial sleep deprivation rather than disturbance in the sleep itself.

Several theories have been proposed concerning the function of sleep. The fact that every living creature sleeps clearly points to sleep being a necessity of life. Indeed when total sleep deprivation is experimentally induced in animals, it results in death within approximately 10 days. In humans, there is a very rare prion disease resulting in gradually increasing sleep loss which culminates in a total loss of sleep and death within a few months (fatal familial insomnia, see later). The exact function of sleep is, however, yet to be determined. Table 4 lists several theories regarding the function of sleep.

As mentioned earlier, sleep has been perceived as a period during which hypnotoxins accumulating during wakefulness are detoxified. Constantin Von Economo, the celebrated discoverer of encephalitis lethargica, postulated that sleep starts once the levels of hypnotoxins reach a critical level, which affects a specific brain centre that is susceptible to these hypnotoxins. Once this brain centre is affected, sleep

Table 4 The possible function of sleep

Protective behaviour
Energy conservation
Brain restoration
Homoeostasis
Improving immune function, temperature regulation

spreads across the brain by pavlovian inhibition. Once detoxification of hypnotoxins is complete, sleep ends. The two-process sleep theory that relied on this assumption has put major emphasis on slow-wave sleep (SWS), as reflecting the brain process responsible for this detoxification. The fact that SWS linearly increases with the duration of previous wakefulness, and exponentially decreases during sleep, supports this position.

Behavioural adaptation sleep theory posits that sleep evolved in order to enforce behavioural quiescence during the dark periods, when organisms may be exposed to better equipped predators. The Benington/Heler theory suggests that sleep fulfils energy conservation purposes. This theory is supported by the findings that during wakefulness the levels of energy in the brain decrease (ATP, glycogen, adenosine), and re-increase during sleep. During sleep itself, the energy expenditure is reduced by 15–20%, and oxygen consumption decreases.

The restorative theory suggests that sleep is a time of restoration and growth for the body and brain. The finding that sleep increases after rigorous exercise supports this theory, as does the observation that growth hormone is mainly released during sleep, especially during deep sleep. Others suggested that sleep is essential for brain processing and organizing the large amounts of input gathered during the day, in a fashion that will allow recollection and use of these data in the future. REM sleep may play a specific role in this regard (see later).

Experimental data suggest that sleep may also be related to temperature regulation and immune defence mechanisms.

The multiplicity of sleep theories most probably indicates that sleep does not have a single function. To cite Kleitman's now famous dictum, when asked what is the function of sleep, his response was: 'Tell me first what is the function of wakefulness and then I will tell you what is the function of sleep.' Most probably as yet unknown functions of sleep still await discovery.

Sleep architecture

The ultradian organization of sleep is in cycles, each of which lasts approximately 1 hour in infants and small children, and 1.5 hours in adults. Every cycle consists of various stages of sleep, usually progressing from stage 1 to 3–4 and culminating in REM sleep. The relative quantity of each of the sleep stages changes as the night progresses. Figure 2 demonstrates a typical 'hypnogram' over a 7.5-hour sleep period. As can be seen, the percentage of SWS is highest in the first sleep cycle, whereas most of the REM sleep is seen towards the morning. The relative part of REM sleep in each sleep cycle increases as the night progresses. Moreover, the density of eye movements in each REM sleep, which most probably reflects the intensity of activation of an endogenous REM sleep generator, also increased as the night progresses.

In reality the sleep cycles are not always complete and frequently in

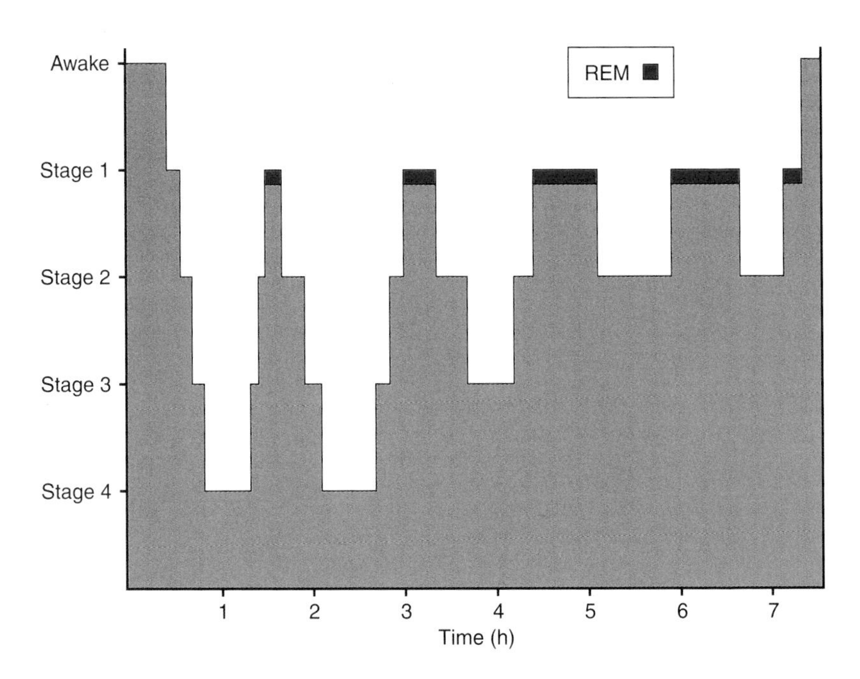

Figure 2 *The characteristics of sleep architecture over a 7.5-hour sleep period.*

some cycles not all sleep stages occur. Commonly, there are short awakenings between sleep cycles, and it is also not unusual to experience some brief arousals within the sleep cycles themselves. When summarizing the relative portion of each of the sleep stages across the night (see Table 3), the following picture emerges: SWS and REM sleep each account for 20% of the total sleep time, and the rest is made up of stages 2 and 1. These percentages change with various conditions such as age (see Table 3), after sleep deprivation, stress, exercise, mood changes and various pathological conditions (see later).

REM sleep – characteristics and function

Rapid eye movement sleep is a unique state of consciousness. It was discovered by Eugene Aserinsky and Nathaniel Kleitman (1953) at the University of Chicago, and has been the subject of extensive research ever since. Its unique physiological and psychological characteristics have led investigators to call it by different names. As EEG activity during REM sleep resembles that of wakefulness it has been called desynchronized sleep, or paradoxical sleep, and because it is associated with dreaming in humans it is often called dreaming sleep. The most commonly used name, however, has remained REM sleep. Indeed the prolific rapid eye movements are the hallmark of this sleep stage. The main characteristics of REM sleep are shown in Table 5.

The confluence of physiological events during REM sleep is rather unique. First, as mentioned before, the EEG is very similar to that of wakefulness, with low-amplitude fast activity, and eye movement activity that is indistinguishable from that in wakefulness. Second, there is evidence of an increased energy expenditure by the brain. Third, in sharp contrast to brain wave and eye movement activation, skeletal muscles are atonic, which is thought to be a protective mechanism to prevent acting out dreams (as may happen in REM behavioural disorder, see Chapter 9). The eye movements probably reflect visualization of dreams, as best indicated by their absence in congenitally blind people as opposed to their presence in acquired blindness. REM sleep is also

Table 5 Characteristics of REM sleep

Arousal threshold	Relatively deep sleep. Increased arousal threshold to various stimuli
EEG	Desynchronized (low amplitude with high-mixed frequency, similar to that of stage 1)
EOG	Rapid eye movements (visualization of vivid dreams, which are characteristic of this stage)
EMG	Absent; effective paralysis – atonia of skeletal muscles
Energy consumption	Augmented metabolism and oxygen consumption by the brain, leading to increased brain temperature in humans
Cardiovascular	Variable blood pressure, more variable pulse rate, change in blood flow distribution (↑ to the brain)
Breathing	Less rhythmic; increased respiratory variability; decreased chemosensitivity
Autonomic nervous system	Increased sympathetic tone, relatively diminished parasympathetic tone
Other physiological phenomena	Penile erection in men (increased vaginal blood flow in women)
Consciousness	In humans, awakening from REM sleep is associated with dreaming

characterized by penile erection in men and vaginal blood engorgement in women, making the meaning of a 'unique' state become clear.

In contrast with the non-REM sleep stages, which are characterized by parasympathetic dominance, REM sleep is associated with intense sympathetic activation. This is manifested by an increase in heart and respiratory rates, as well as in their variability, and an increase in peripheral vasoconstriction and systemic blood pressure. Furthermore, the sensitivity of the respiratory control mechanisms to hypercapnia and hypoxia in this stage is diminished, resulting in prolonged apnoeic events and profound arterial oxygen desaturation in sleep apnoea patients (see later). Penile erection, mediated by parasympathetic activation, stands out during REM sleep, on the background of sympathetic dominance. The penile erection seen in REM sleep has important clinical implications because it can distinguish between psychogenic and organic impotence. The existence of REM-related penile erection rules out organic causes of impotence.

Despite extensive research spanning almost half a century, the exact function of REM is far from being understood. Table 6 lists several theories regarding the function of REM sleep.

The main findings from studies (of animals and humans) addressing the issue of the function of REM sleep can be briefly summarized as follows:

- REM sleep deprivation disrupts learning of complex or new tasks.
- Successful learning during wakefulness results in increased REM during the next sleep.
- Without REM sleep the recollection of newly learned material is impaired.

There is experimental evidence supporting the possible role of REM sleep in learning and memory consolidation processes. Thus, sleep episodes after learning of new materials consist of increased numbers of REM sleep episodes, prolongation of the first REM period and increases in REM density. However, that said, certain people demonstrate marked decreases in (or even absence of) REM sleep, yet they do not show any clear impairment of neurocognitive functioning.

One example of this phenomenon is patients on REM-suppressing

Table 6 The possible functions of REM sleep and dreaming
Consolidation of memory and processing newly learned material
Stimulation to the brain
Solving daytime problems and conflicts

medications such as antidepressants. An even more robust example is a patient studied in our laboratory several times after a brain injury that resulted in almost total absence of REM sleep. We studied him in the sleep laboratory for more than 10 nights and found more than a 95% suppression of REM sleep. This patient has shown no evidence of deterioration in his cognitive or mental functions over the last 15 years. It is difficult to reconcile the theories implicating REM sleep in memory and learning processes with our observations in this unique individual (and in those on antidepressants).

A different theory proposes that REM functions as an endogenous source of brain stimulation that at times is needed for brain maturation. Although it is difficult to test this theory empirically, there is some indirect supportive evidence. First, REM sleep occupies most of the sleep in newborns, and gradually decreases with age. Furthermore, its amount is even larger in pre-term infants whose nervous system is immature. The theory does not provide an explanation, however, for why REM sleep persists throughout life, long after the central nervous system has matured. Michel Jouvet, whose studies greatly enhanced our understanding of the neural substrates mediating sleep and REM sleep, suggested that REM sleep is essential for training central neural networks related to instinctive behaviours. He showed in cats that, once the neural system responsible for the REM-related postural atonia has a lesion, sleeping cats periodically displayed a specific repertoire of instinctive behaviours that resembled fighting and exploring, which Jouvet attributed to REM-related activation of neural networks related to instincts. It should also be pointed out that smiling in the human newborn, which is also an instinctive behaviour, was reported to appear for the first time during REM sleep.

In conclusion, the function of REM sleep, which has challenged the imagination of sleep researchers ever since its first description in 1953, is still an enigma. Recent studies utilizing advanced imaging techniques such as positron emission tomography (PET) scanning and functional magnetic resonance imaging (MRI) promise to unveil some of its mystery.

Sleep–wake cycles

In spite of the ubiquitous periodic nature of sleep and wakefulness, recognition of the sleep–wake cycle as a biological rhythm controlled by brain oscillators has been slow to come. Until the 1960s, sleep was mostly conceptualized within the framework of homoeostatic principles. During sleep, energy or essential brain or bodily ingredients, depleted during waking, were thought to be restored. A complementary view posited the accumulation of toxic substances during wakefulness which are detoxified or removed from circulation during sleep. The immediate cause of sleep was sought in the production of these hypnotoxins that inhibit brain activities.

The initial experimental results that point to the sleep–wake rhythm not being passively controlled by the environment, or solely responding to accumulated wake time, came from studies in which sleep was completely eliminated. Keeping individuals awake for prolonged periods of time revealed that, although sleep pressure monotonically increased throughout the deprivation period, it also exhibited pronounced rhythms that covered almost 24 h, with peak alertness during the afternoon and peak sleepiness during the night. Enforcing constant posture on sleep-deprived participants, in addition to uniform and well-controlled lighting and feeding schedules – a procedure termed the 'constant routine' – did not eliminate the sleepiness cycle.

Early studies that investigated the effect of sleep displacement also supported the concept of an endogenous cycle. The most prominent effect of sleep inversion was a significant increase in wakefulness, particularly towards the end of sleep. This effect, which persisted throughout the experiment, was at the expense of REM sleep, which was shifted towards an earlier time in the sleep period. Field studies of shift workers and long-haul aeroplane travellers reached similar conclusions. Displacing sleep from its normal timing has generally been associated with transient insomnia, for at least a few days after the shift (see later).

Direct evidence supporting the endogenous origin of the sleep–wake rhythms was provided in studies in which individuals were isolated from all possible time cues that could potentially affect their rhythmic behaviour. In such a 'time-free environment', sleep–wake rhythms lengthened to approximately 25 h. Only recently was it discovered that the lengthening of the period by 1 h in isolation was probably an artefact of the experimental conditions and that the period of the endogenous sleep–wake cycle is longer than 24 h by no more than 10 minutes. Environmental light, including ordinary indoor light, is the most important factor that entrains the endogenous biological rhythm to the geophysical light–dark cycle.

Thus, the timing of sleep is determined by the combination of at least three factors: homoeostatic drive to sleep which increases as a function of elapsed wake time, circadian cycle in sleep propensity and behavioural influences.

Ontogenesis of sleep (changes with age)

Age greatly influences all aspects of sleep: its quantity, timing, continuity and architecture. The most recent data suggest that well-differentiated behavioural states can be recognized in humans for the first time *in utero*, from the beginning of the third trimester of pregnancy. Preterm babies born at the same gestational age demonstrate similar behavioural states as those *in utero* at equivalent gestational age. The first behavioural state to appear is REM sleep. In early ontogenesis, REM sleep is called active sleep because of the numerous small movements and twitches that characterize this state at this age. Active sleep is the predominant behavioural state, accounting for about 60% of sleep in the newborn, and rapidly decreases to about 30–35% at age 3 months. It then gradually decreases to the adult level of approximately 20% between 2 and 6 years of age. The initial decrease in active sleep occurs mainly as a result of fewer episodes rather than shorter episodes.

The second stage to be seen is NREM (quiet) sleep, which is characterized in fetuses by discontinuous EEG (i.e. 'gaps' between EEG activity), and in newborns by an EEG pattern of trace alternance. This pattern disappears at approximately 3–6 weeks of age. At 6–9 weeks, sleep spindles and K-complexes can be recognized. Quiet (NREM) sleep can be divided into the four adult-like sleep stages at the age of 2–3 months. Wakefulness is the last behaviour to appear during pregnancy. Fetuses sleep most of the time, and newborns sleep approximately 16 hours per day.

The circadian rhythm also matures in the first few months of life. At birth, melatonin, which is a hormone responsible for entraining the circadian sleep–wake rhythm to the environmental light–dark cycle (see later), cannot be detected and circadian rhythm cannot be recognized. Sleep–wake cycles are approximately 4 hours, consisting of mainly sleep and some wakefulness. At birth, there is no difference between day and night in terms of sleep–wake distribution. It takes about 3–4 months for the circadian rhythm to consolidate, and thus at age 4 months infants can sleep 6–7 hours continuously during the night, and stay awake for increasingly longer periods during the day. Up to the age of 2 years, toddlers may nap two to three times every day, which decreases to one nap by the age of 6. After this sleep assumes the adult monophasic characteristic, although napping is not uncommon in adults as well.

Sleep in children is very 'deep' with extremely high arousal thresholds. This characteristic is gradually modified over time, together with the decrease in the amplitude of EEG δ waves. The δ amplitude may be as high as 300–500 μV in children, decrease to 100–150 μV in adults, and hardly exceed 75–100 μV in elderly people. The total time of sleep also decreases from childhood to adulthood, although commonly during puberty individuals may temporarily dramatically increase their total sleep time.

Whether elderly people need less sleep is controversial. Previously, it was thought that they do, and it has been suggested that the reason may be a reduction in the number of neurons and amount of brain tissue. However, recent research revealed that, in fact, elderly people need the same amount of sleep as adults. Their reduced nocturnal sleep time was explained by napping during the day and an alteration in the circadian oscillator regulating sleep–wake behaviour. It appears that there is a tendency towards an advance of the circadian phase of sleepiness relative to the temperature rhythm in elderly people, which may explain their tendency to early morning awakening. In addition, as stated, the δ wave amplitude decreases in elderly people, and the arousal threshold decreases too, which makes them vulnerable to environmental noises. Sleep in elderly people may also be affected by medical illnesses and/or usage of medications (discussed later).

In addition, the pineal body, which is responsible for melatonin production and secretion and tends to be calcified with ageing, may be associated with a decrease in melatonin production and in circadian rhythm abnormalities. Inadequate exposure to light–dark cycles also may be a contributing factor. Although controversial, melatonin replacement therapy was reported to have beneficial effects in these cases (see later). Finally, the normal alertness during the day also changes with age. Children are typically 'hyper-alert', with average sleep onset latency (SOL) (based on the Multiple Sleep Latency Test – MSLT) score of around 20–25 minutes compared with 15 minutes in adults. Thus, when dealing with sleep disorders it is always important to take age into consideration, because it has important effects on sleep.

Sleep deprivation

Sleep deprivation can come in many forms. It can result from brief total sleep deprivation, such as skipping a sleep period because of a night job, from chronic partial sleep loss or from a combination of both. Most people need 7–9 hours of sleep per day (more during childhood). In most Western societies, people are pushing the limits of this sleep–wake balance. They extend their wakefulness, at the expense of adequate sleep. This partial sleep deprivation is characteristic of some specific occupations, such as physicians, long-distance truck drivers and others. Table 7 summarizes the effects of sleep deprivation.

Obviously the sleep-deprived individual is sleepy, although sometimes the behavioural manifestation is paradoxically hyperactivity, especially in children. Other behavioural and mood changes can also be observed such as irritability, nervousness, violence, depression, mania, bipolar behaviour, etc. Functional impairment has been noted in practically every experiment investigating sleep deprivation. Some of the effects of sleep deprivation may be ameliorated with stimulants such as caffeine

Table 7 Consequences of sleep deprivation

Behavioural	Sleepiness	(Both subjective and objective)
	Mood changes	Depression/mania
	Irritability, nervousness	Can turn to violence
Cognitive	Impairment of function	Newly learned skills
		Short-term memory
		Complex tasks
		Slow reaction time
Neurological	Mild and quickly reversible	Nystagmus, tremor, ptosis, slurred speech, increased reflexes (gag, tendon), increased sensitivity to pain
Biochemical	Increased metabolic rate Increased thyroid activity Insulin resistance	In animals, decreased weight despite increased caloric intake (secondary to increased energy requirement?)
Others	Hypothermia, perhaps immune function impairment	

(e.g. subjective sleepiness), but only to some extent, and not all (e.g. temporal memory remains impaired without any effect of stimulants). The somatic effects of sleep deprivation presented in Table 7 (i.e. neurological, biochemical and 'others') are very mild and quickly reversible with recovery sleep. Furthermore, most of these data are based on only a few studies, and some of the findings could not be reproduced.

The threshold at which symptoms and signs of sleep deprivation are observed obviously depends on the amount of sleep loss, as well as on factors such as motivation, personality and nutritional state. For this reason, various studies have revealed conflicting results. Some researchers believe that most normal young adults who sleep 8 hours every 24 hours can tolerate quite well chronic sleep loss of 2–3 hours per day, i.e. sleeping 5–6 hours every 24 hours. When highly motivated, they may be able to live with such sleep deprivation for several weeks without demonstrating any obvious daytime functional compromise. Others, however, have shown that young adults who sleep regularly 7–8 hours every day significantly improve their performance with an increase in their sleep time. Thus, it seems that sleep deprivation often makes an impact, although it may be masked to some extent on occasions.

Another important question is whether the amount of compensatory recovery sleep corresponds to the amount of sleep loss during sleep deprivation periods. Current data suggest that this may not be the case. It has been shown that a recovery sleep period of only 8 h appears to be adequate to regain baseline performance levels after short-term sleep deprivation. It has also been demonstrated that, after chronic partial sleep deprivation, baseline levels of performance may return following shorter compensatory sleep time than the actual sleep loss. Sleep architecture during recovery sleep is characterized by increased SWS. Moreover, δ activity during recovery sleep is of higher amplitude than baseline sleep, which implicates deep SWS as responsible for the restorative function of sleep.

chapter 2

Systemic function during normal sleep

The sleep–wake cycle is an output of the central nervous system, but may affect almost every other somatic system. In some phenomena, it is difficult to distinguish between sleep effects and circadian effects (i.e. nocturnal), because in the normal population, on whom most of the studies took place, sleep occurs during the night period. Some studies have addressed this issue, and reported direct effects of sleep or circadian timing on the various physiological systems. In this chapter we briefly review these systems.

The neuromuscular system

As stated previously, during sleep the central nervous system (CNS) remains active and in fact determines the behavioural state in an active process. It is beyond the scope of this book to go into details of the function of the various regions of the brain in the different sleep stages. Briefly, it is generally believed that the cerebral cortex does not possess an intrinsic mechanism for its own activation, and thus the maintenance of wakefulness requires ascending excitatory input from the subcortical structures and brain stem.

The major regions responsible for wakefulness include the reticular formation (projections from various regions), basal forebrain (cholinergic), locus coeruleus (noradrenergic), dorsal raphe (serotoninergic) and the posterior hypothalamus (which includes the tuberomammillary nucleus – histaminergic, dorsolateral area – hypocretin/orexin-mediated, dopaminergic A11 region and glutamatergic neurons). The main region responsible for sleep is the ventrolateral preoptic area (VLPO, GABA-ergic where GABA is γ-aminobutyric acid), whereas the major regions responsible for REM sleep are the cholinergic laterodorsal tegmental (LDT) nucleus and the pedunculopontine tegmental nucleus (PPT). Therefore, very roughly it can be stated that the predominant neurotransmitters participating in the maintenance of wakefulness are acetylcholine, norepinephrine (noradrenaline) and serotonin, during sleep GABA, and during rapid eye movement (REM) sleep again acetylcholine. This is summarized in Table 8. Obviously, this is a brief and simplified summary because many other neurotransmitters play a role as well (e.g. glutamate, aspartate, hypocretin/orexin, histamine, adenosine, galanine, substance P, etc.).

As discussed elsewhere (see Figure 1 and Table 2), the summary of the neuronal activities from various regions can be recorded by electrodes placed on the scalp (EEG). The term 'EEG desynchronized' is usually used to describe the low-amplitude, mixed-frequency (usually fast) activity seen during REM sleep. The sleep spindle, which is a synchronized type of activity characterized by the appearance of approximately 1 s of 12–14 Hz waves, originates in the thalamus, and marks sleep (it cannot be detected during wakefulness). Another major synchronized EEG is δ activity (slow wave high amplitude), which probably originates in the

Table 8 The predominant neurotransmitters in the various behavioural states

Behavioural state	*Acetylcholine*	*Norepinephrine (noradrenaline)*	*Serotonin (5HT)*
Wake	++	++	++
Non-REM sleep	–	+	+
REM sleep	++	–	–

cortex and marks deep sleep. The rest of the major rhythms important in staging of the behavioural state are the α rhythm (originates in the occipital cortex) and the θ rhythm (originates in the hippocampus).

Unlike the CNS, the peripheral nervous system (PNS) seems to be 'less active' during sleep and thus deep tendon reflexes are inhibited during sleep (e.g. the patellar reflex). This phenomenon may be one of the reasons for the development of sleep apnoea syndrome, because during sleep we lose the protective reflex of activation of the upper airway muscles in response to negative pressure (see later). From the muscular point of view, there is gradual muscle relaxation as sleep deepens, reaching virtual atonia of the skeletal muscles during REM sleep. In several pathological conditions, muscles remain active during sleep, and these are discussed in Chapters 5 and 9. It should also be mentioned that the process of hyperpolarization of the anterior horn in the spinal cord (α motorneuron) matures only at 3–4 months of age, so in neonates and infants some muscle twitches are very common during REM sleep.

The autonomic nervous system

When discussing the function of the autonomic nervous system (ANS) during sleep, we should distinguish between the effect of sleep and the effect of the circadian rhythm on the ANS, because both may have substantial effects. Moreover, the effects of both on the ANS may be differential (i.e. different results in the various organs innervated by this system). The activity of the ANS may be evaluated directly by measuring neuronal outflow of sympathetic fibres, or by the effects on target organs such as the heart, vascular system, pupils, etc. It is beyond the scope of this book to go into details of the normal physiology of the ANS in the various behavioural states and/or circadian phases, so the following represents only a brief summary of the main findings on this issue. The reader is referred to some specific papers which review this topic specifically (Horner, Parmeggiani, Hedner).

Generally, direct measurements of sympathetic nerve outflow in animals reveal that there is a slight decrease in sympathetic activity with the transition from wakefulness to sleep. This may be diminished further with the transition to tonic REM sleep, although it may be substantially increased during phasic REM sleep. Conversely, it seems that parasympathetic activity increases with the transition from wakefulness to sleep, and further increases or persists unchanged during REM sleep. This may be evident from the myosis seen in animals during sleep (relative to wakefulness), although, again, during bursts of eye movements representing phasic REM, phasic dilatation of the pupils may be seen. By measuring muscle sympathetic nerve activity (microneurography of peroneal nerve in humans), it seems that sympathetic activation decreases as non-REM (NREM) sleep deepens, and increases during REM sleep. However, when sympathetic activity is recorded in other sympathetic nerves (e.g. the renal nerve, which is technically very difficult and can be done only in animals), the changes in sympathetic activity with transition from wakefulness to sleep seems to be minimal. Although the bradycardia seen during sleep compared with wakefulness (see later) can be explained by a decrease in sympathetic activation, it seems more likely that it results from increased parasympathetic activation because it can also be seen in sympathectomized animals. Table 9 summarizes the general changes in the ANS with behavioural state.

Another method of evaluating autonomic function is by examining the beat-to-beat variations of the heart rate (heart rate variability or HRV). By this method, the parasympathetic system's output is in the high-frequency range (HF), whereas sympathetic activity is in the low-frequency range (LF), as illustrated in Figure 3.

Studies that have examined the changes in HRV as a function of the circadian rhythm (excluding the effects of sleep) very carefully, revealed that at around the temperature nadir, about 4 am, there is peak parasympathetic activation. This may explain the high incidence of asthmatic attacks at this time (the increased parasympathetic tone results in bronchoconstriction). Sympathetic activation may be less affected by the circadian rhythm, although ongoing studies are investigating this issue.

Table 9 The effect of behavioural state on ANS activity

Transition	*Wakefulness to NREM sleep*	*NREM to REM sleep*	*Comments*
Sympathetic	Decrease	Differential and variable:	
		Decrease in renal	
		Increase in muscles	
		Decrease to heart (tonic)	Increase (phasic)
Parasympathetic	Increase	Unchanged or increased	Variable in REM

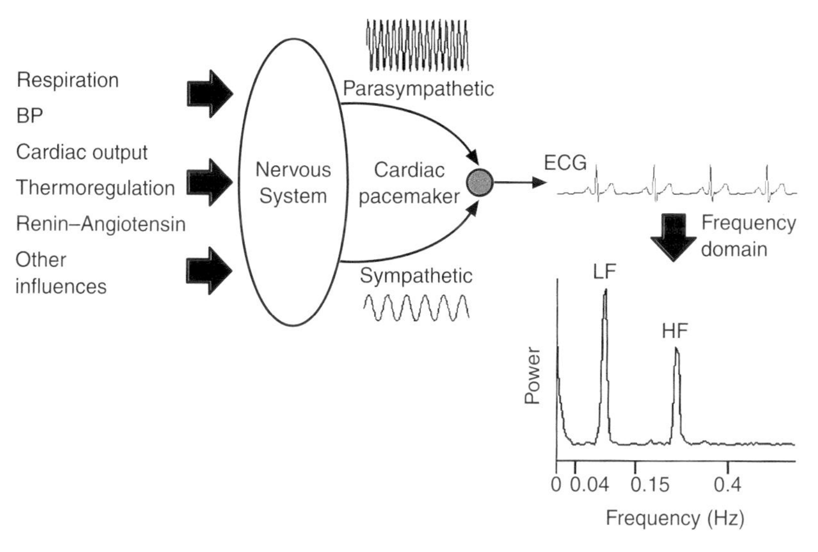

Figure 3 *Heart rate variability and the autonomic nervous system. BP, blood pressure; HF, high frequency; HRV, heart rate variability; LF, low frequency.*

The cardiovascular system

The cardiovascular system is under the effect of the ANS, so the changes reflect the balance between sympathetic and parasympathetic activities. NREM sleep is generally associated with reductions in heart rate (HR) and blood pressure (BP) compared with established wakefulness. Tonic REM sleep is associated with further decreases, whereas phasic REM sleep events produce characteristic phasic increase in HR and BP. The net effect of REM sleep is thus variable, and largely depends on the proportion of phasic (vs tonic) REM episodes.

As stroke volume is only minimally affected by sleep, cardiac output (CO) largely follows that of HR, and thus decreases with the transition from wakefulness to sleep, and further decreases with the transition to REM sleep. The decrement of BP from wakefulness to sleep results mainly from the decrement in CO, because the total peripheral resistance (TPR) only minimally changes with the wake–sleep transition. During REM sleep, there is a decrease in TPR, which is indicative of net vasodilatation. We found that REM sleep is associated with digital vasoconstriction, which may result from the decrement in CO; this can also explain the overall decrement in BP during REM sleep. Studies have revealed that the vascular changes during REM sleep are differential, e.g. there is vasodilatation in the mesenteric and renal vascular beds, but vasoconstriction in the iliac and skeletal muscle circulations.

Skeletal muscle vasculature is also thought to play an important role in producing the phasic increases in BP that typically occur during phasic REM events (transient vasoconstrictions). These data are summarized in Table 10.

As a result of the different changes seen during tonic versus phasic REM, the net effect is usually high variability of HR, CO, BP and TPR overall during REM sleep. This phenomenon is also characteristic for the respiratory system (see below).

Table 10 The effect of behavioural state on the cardiovascular system

Transition	*Wakefulness to NREM sleep*	*NREM to tonic REM sleep*	*Phasic REM sleep*
Heart rate	Decreases	Decreases	Increases
Cardiac output	Decreases	Decreases	Increases
Blood pressure	Decreases	Decreases	Increases
Total peripheral resistance	Minimal changes	Decreases	Increases

Respiration

The control of breathing during wakefulness responds to three major stimuli: chemical (the arterial partial pressures Pa_{O_2}, Pa_{CO_2}, and pH), mechanical (receptors in the lung and chest wall) and behavioural (cortical). During sleep, behavioural influences are absent, and ventilation becomes totally involuntary. With the transition from wakefulness to sleep, ventilation usually decreases. During NREM sleep, respiration is regular, with lower tidal volume and respiratory rate (compared with wakefulness), which leads to a decline in minute ventilation (falls by 8–15% compared with wakefulness). Thus, sleep is associated with a mild increase in end-tidal CO_2 ($ETCO_2$) and decrease in O_2 saturation. This decrease in ventilation, in combination with the supine position and a decrease in intercostal muscle tone, results in a decrease in functional residual capacity (FRC). Furthermore, a sleep-related decrease in upper airway muscle tone and lung volume results in a marked increase in upper airway resistance.

During REM sleep, breathing is irregular, with variable respiratory rate and tidal volume, and frequent central apnoeas. Inhibition of tonic activity of the intercostal muscles results in a further decline in FRC. Hypotonia of the upper airway muscles in the presence of unchanged diaphragmatic contractions during REM sleep predisposes individuals to obstructive apnoeas. Tidal volume, respiratory rate and minute ventilation, however, remain unchanged (on average) in REM sleep compared with NREM sleep.

The ventilatory response to chemical stimuli is also state dependent. The ventilatory response to both hypoxia and hypercapnia falls during sleep in adult humans, and declines further in REM sleep. Finally, sleep modifies the ventilatory response to added inspiratory resistance. Although inspiratory resistance load during wakefulness results in increased inspiratory time and relatively unchanged ventilation, sleep blunts this response and ventilation falls in response to loading. We have recently shown that this fall in ventilation is greater in men than in women, as a result of higher upper airway resistance in men (rather than sex-related differences in central respiratory drive). Table 11 shows

Table 11 Average normal adult ventilation variables across behavioural states

	Awake	*NREM*	*REM*
Tidal volume (ml)	500	450	450
Respiratory rate (/min)	14	13	13
Minute ventilation (l/min)	7	6	6
Upper airway resistance (cmH_2O/l per s)	2	5	6
Hypoxic ventilatory response (l/min per % SaO_2)	0.7	0.6	0.4
Hypercapnic ventilatory response (l/min per mmHg)	2.5	0.8	0.7

some average normal values for the respiratory variables during the various behavioural states, driven by our studies and those of others performed on normal young adult volunteers.

The gastrointestinal system

It is quite surprising that the effect of sleep and circadian rhythm on gastrointestinal function has been only minimally studied, despite the relatively high incidence of nocturnal symptoms in gastrointestinal disorders, e.g. in shift workers, gastrointestinal complaints are among the most frequent symptoms observed clinically. Nocturnal epigastric pain (peptic ulcer) or heartburn may result in difficulties falling asleep and maintaining sleep. One reason for the increased incidence of heartburn during sleep is the postural change from standing to supine sleeping. However, sleep may have some other influences resulting in increased sleep-related gastrointestinal symptoms. First, sleep is normally relatively free of episodes of gastro-oesophageal reflux. However, whenever such an event occurs during sleep, it is associated with substantial prolongation of the acid clearance time from the oesophagus. This occurs as a result of a delay in the conscious response to acid in the oesophagus during sleep, and the need for awakening in order to transport the acid from the distal oesophagus to the stomach. In addition, salivary flow stops with the onset of sleep and therefore also contributes to slower neutralization of an acidic oesophagus. Sleep depresses the frequency of swallows, which contributes to slower clearance of acid from the oesophagus (reduced primary peristalsis).

Whether sleep changes the competence of the lower oesophageal sphincter is unknown. It has been shown that most gastro-oesophageal reflux events occur as a result of a spontaneous decline in the pressure of the lower oesophageal sphincter, whereas others occur secondary to increased intra-abdominal pressure. The latter may result from postural changes during sleep and/or obstructive sleep-disordered breathing (see Chapter 4). The peak in acid secretion in the stomach occurs between 10 pm and 2 am, which probably reflects the increased parasympathetic (vagal) tone, as 24-h gastric pH measurements subsequent to vagotomy do not exhibit a clear circadian rhythm.

The effects of sleep on other gastrointestinal functions, such as gastric emptying, intestinal tone, intestinal/colonic motility and liver/bile function, were either minimally studied or revealed conflicting results.

One interesting concept of sleep and gastrointestinal system is the potential effect of the gastrointestinal system on sleep. Most people experience sleepiness after a heavy meal (postprandial sleepiness). Several mechanisms can explain this fascinating phenomenon. First, a heavy meal can induce re-distribution of the blood supply, with increased abdominal blood flow at the expense of brain blood flow. However, interestingly, cortical synchronization can be induced by inflating a balloon in the small bowel (i.e. causing distension) or by electrical stimulation of the bowel, without food at all. Thus, alternative explanations include either afferent nerve fibre input from the small intestine to the CNS (via the splanchnic nerve), or the effect of gastrointestinal hormones (e.g. cholecystokinin).

In conclusion, there may be a variety of sleep/circadian effects on the gastrointestinal tract, but clearly more studies are needed for better understanding of the relationship between sleep and the gastrointestinal system.

Body temperature

Body temperature varies throughout the day in a regular rhythmic pattern. The circadian cycle in humans usually peaks during the late afternoon or evening hours, and reaches a nadir in the early morning hours. The cycle in body temperature, which is under the control of the biological clock residing in the suprachiasmatic nucleus (SCN) of the hypothalamus, is modified by sleep but is not dependent on it. Circadian cycles in temperature are clearly evident during prolonged sleep deprivation periods, and inversion of the sleep–wake cycle, as seen in shift workers or jet lag, does not result in an immediate reversal of the body temperature cycle. Sleep, however, modifies the cycle by decreasing body temperature further, which is superimposed on the circadian pattern. There is a complex relationship between the timing and duration of sleep and the circadian rhythm in body temperature. When sleep starts during the late afternoon peak in body temperature, it is short and disrupted, whereas sleep occurring on the downward slope of the body temperature rhythm, which is the time when sleep normally occurs, is prolonged and more restful.

There are data to suggest that sleep may be essential for maintaining core body temperature within biologically functional limits. Prolonged sleep deprivation in rats caused a profound and lethal hypothermia, which was associated with abnormal responses to thermal challenges. Yet, there are no comparable data in humans.

The endocrine system

Daily oscillations characterize the release of almost every hormone. The daily profile for each hormone is the product of complex interactions of the output of the circadian pacemaker (SCN), changes in behaviour, light exposure, neuroendocrine feedback mechanisms, sex, age and the sleep–wakefulness state. Meals and exercise may also cause some changes in hormonal levels. Each endocrine system is differentially affected by these factors. This chapter reviews mainly hormonal systems that are affected predominantly by sleep (e.g. growth hormone or GH) or those that are affected by the circadian rhythm but relatively unaffected by sleep (e.g. melatonin and cortisol).

To distinguish between the sleep effect on a hormone and that of the circadian rhythm, the constant routine method was developed. In this method, the sleep–wake schedule and its associated posture, lighting, meals, social contacts and level of external stimuli are dissociated from the usual time of sleep. In this protocol, human volunteers remain awake in a semi-recumbent position in dim, indoor room light, receiving frequent, small meals for 30–60 hours. Therefore, the evoked effects of changes in posture, sleep–wake state, meal size and lighting conditions are minimized across circadian phases. Thus, measuring hormone levels during a constant routine protocol reveals the circadian effects only, without the influence of sleep, although this protocol does cause cumulative sleep deprivation. This chapter focuses on circadian and sleep-dependent regulation of the most widely studied and relevant hormones.

Melatonin

Melatonin is a neurohormone produced by the pineal gland, normally secreted exclusively during darkness. Recent research has shown that melatonin has a dual effect: sleep promotion and circadian pacemaker phase shift. Its primary function is to control the circadian rhythm and entrainment to the light–dark cycle, but it also has a mild hypnotic effect and thus increases the propensity for sleep. In addition, it may have a role in the biological regulation of mood, and perhaps reproduction, tumour growth and ageing.

The circadian rhythm in melatonin production and secretion is under the control of the biological clock (SCN), and is synchronized with the environmental light–dark cycle. Photic information from the retina is transmitted to the pineal gland through the SCN and the sympathetic nervous system. The neural input to the gland is norepinephrine (noradrenaline), and the output is melatonin. The synthesis and release of melatonin are inhibited by light. Melatonin secretion normally increases soon after the onset of darkness, peaks in the middle of the night

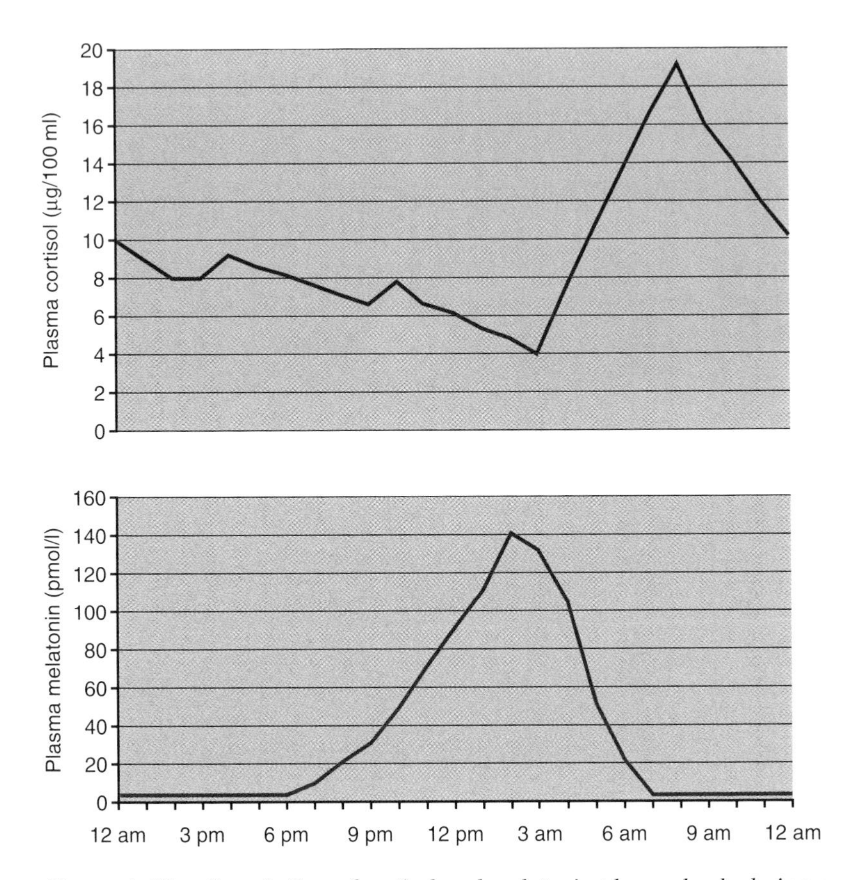

Figure 4 *Circadian rhythm of cortisol and melatonin plasma levels during a constant routine in normal adult. Neither melatonin nor cortisol are affected by sleep, and their secretion reflects primarily the circadian rhythm.*

(2–4 am) and gradually falls during the second half of the night (Figure 4). The melatonin profile monitored on a constant routine is almost indistinguishable from that recorded under entrained conditions, suggesting that the absence of the nocturnal sleep episode has little effect on the daily profile. Therefore, melatonin is frequently used as a marker of the circadian phase.

Melatonin secretion is not affected by the sex of the subject or, in women, by the menstrual cycle. It is, however, affected by age. Infants younger than 3 months secrete very little melatonin. With an appropriate exposure to light and dark cycles, melatonin secretion increases and acquires its circadian profile, starting at age 4–6 months. The peak nocturnal concentrations of melatonin are highest at the age of 1–3 years (approximately 1400 pmol/l), after which they decline gradually. In normal young adults the average nocturnal peak melatonin level is 260 pmol/l. In some elderly people, there is a tendency for the pineal gland to calcify, and melatonin secretion may decrease. If there is an associated insomnia, we have found that supplemental melatonin may improve their sleep.

Cortisol

Cortisol is a steroid secreted by the adrenal cortex (zona fasciculata), in a pulsatile fashion. It is the principal glucocorticoid, which affects the metabolism of most tissues. It has mainly catabolic effects, resulting in increased degradation of proteins, mainly in the muscles, skin, connective and adipose tissues. Cortisol, on the other hand, is anabolic in the liver, where it stimulates gluconeogenesis. Cortisol synthesis is regulated primarily by ACTH (adrenocorticotrophic hormone), with cortisol exerting negative feedback on ACTH secretion. Cortisol secretion is under circadian regulation, with the lowest daily levels measured slightly after midnight and the highest daily levels found in the early morning (Figure 4). As cortisol is one of the 'stress hormones', it was initially thought that the morning rise in cortisol level expresses the stress of wake time, or that of REM sleep towards the morning. In fact, later studies have demonstrated that sleep has a very minor effect on cortisol levels. The 24-hour profile of cortisol concentration in people on a regular sleep–wake schedule is very similar to that of those remaining awake throughout the night on a constant routine protocol.

Thus, the circadian clock rather than sleep drives the daily changes in cortisol levels. In fact, the tight regulation of the cortisol rhythm by the circadian pacemaker is one reason why the peak of the cortisol level is frequently used as a marker of circadian phase. Furthermore, one of the potential reasons for the known exacerbation of asthma, stridor or bronchiolitis during the night may be the decline in cortisol levels, and therefore the increase in inflammatory processes in the airway walls.

Careful inspection reveals that the change in cortisol levels throughout the day is caused by changes in pulse amplitude rather than pulse frequency. Sleep itself either poses a modest inhibition of cortisol secretion or does not change it. Awakening, on the other hand, results in a slight increase in cortisol level on top of the circadian increase during wake time.

Finally, as cortisol levels change dramatically with the time of day, it is very important for clinical purposes (for the diagnosis of cortisol excess or deficiency) to measure cortisol levels at the specific time to which the reference levels refer (usually 8 am).

Growth hormone

Growth hormone is a protein with 191 amino acids produced by the anterior pituitary gland. The regulation of GH release is under the control of two hypothalamic hormones. Growth hormone-releasing hormone (GHRH) stimulates, and somatostatin inhibits, GH release. Alternating secretion of GHRH and somatostatin accounts for the rhythmic secretion of GH, which appears to have a dominant 2-hour periodicity.

Growth hormone may act directly on tissues, but in most body organs GH acts through insulin-like growth factor 1 (IGF-1), formerly known as somatomedin C. IGF-1 levels correlate with GH levels. In children, GH is crucial to skeletal development, promoting endochondral ossification, elongation of chondrocyte columns and widening of epiphyseal plates. Many of these growth processes are dependent on local tissue and remote production of IGF-1. GH also increases muscle protein stores and has anabolic effects on body composition. In addition, GH has metabolic effects. Initially, it produces a brief insulin-like response with temporary hypoglycaemia. After about 2 hours, it may result in hyperglycaemia mainly as a result of inhibition of uptake of glucose by muscle and fatty tissue. Finally, GH may also promote the breakdown of triglycerides to free fatty acids (FFAs), which may increase the concentration of FFAs in the blood. The main consequence of the absence of GH in childhood is dwarfism.

As GH is secreted in a pulsatile fashion, and has a relatively short serum half-life (22 min), a single random GH level provides very little information on the total 24-h GH secretion of an individual. The highest levels of GH are achieved during sleep. Although GH levels start to increase in the late evening before the sleep episode begins, it does not have a dominant independent circadian rhythm, and its secretion is rather related to sleep, especially (but not exclusively) to slow wave sleep (SWS). In constant routine protocols, it has been shown that a pulse of GH is more likely to occur at the usual time of sleep onset, whether or not the individual sleeps at that time. However, the secretory episode is smaller than if sleep occurred. There are quite a number of studies supporting the association between SWS and GH secretion. These studies reported that GH secretory bursts closely related to SWS, correlation between δ activity power in the EEG and GH levels, and drugs that promote SWS (γ-hydroxybutyrate) increase GH secretion.

Furthermore, experimentally induced arousals during SWS have reduced the magnitude of GHRH-induced GH secretory pulses. Nevertheless, there are some investigators challenging this tight relationship between SWS and GH secretion. There is consensus, however, that in normal entrained humans the predominant portion of the total 24-h GH release occurs in the first hours of sleep, when SWS is predominant as well. In the absence of sleep during a constant routine protocol, although there is typically a secretory episode of GH near the habitual bed-time, it is markedly reduced in amplitude and is no longer a predominant component of the daily GH profile. Individuals with a free-running circadian rhythm (not entrained to the 24-h clock time), with dissociation between the sleep–wake rhythm and the circadian rhythm, have lower amounts of GH secreted at the start of sleep episodes despite comparable amounts of SWS. This suggests that an interaction between sleep and the circadian pacemaker affects GH secretion, although, again, it appears that the predominant factor is sleep itself and not the circadian rhythm.

As GH release is associated with SWS, it has been suggested that children with sleep disorders and therefore disturbed SWS may have growth retardation. Indeed, it has been shown that children with sleep apnoea have lower levels of IGF-1, associated with the severity of the sleep apnoea. Furthermore, children with psychosocial dwarfism exhibit a decrease in SWS (which is not observed in genetic dwarfism). In addition, certain stressful conditions interfering with sleep, such as depression and other psychosocial problems, are believed to affect GH secretion during sleep. Thus, disturbed SWS may have a clinical role in terms of decreased GH in children. Its clinical role in adults is questionable.

Finally, it should be mentioned that GH secretion is affected by the sex hormones, and differs between the sexes and, in women, it changes with the menstrual cycle. The concentration of GH release at the initial sleep time is much more prominent in men, whereas in women GH pulses are more spread throughout the day and night.

Thyroid-stimulating hormone

Thyroid-stimulating hormone (TSH, thyrotrophin) is another anterior pituitary hormone. Its synthesis and release are stimulated by the hypothalamic TSH-releasing hormone (TRH), and it affects the thyroid gland to release thyroid hormones.

Similar to GH and prolactin (see later), sleep has prominent effects on TSH secretion. Normally, TSH levels peak in the late evening (towards midnight), and decline following the start of the nocturnal sleep episode. This can be logically explained by the lower metabolic rate during sleep, and thus the lower 'need' for the thyroid hormone. However, it has only recently been demonstrated that the nocturnal decline in TSH is a sleep-related inhibitory effect rather than a circadian effect. During a constant routine protocol, TSH levels actually increase at the time of the habitual start of the nocturnal sleep episode, and peak in the middle of the night (approximately 3 am). The circadian rhythm in TSH levels includes a rise in the evening, higher levels during the beginning of the night, and lower levels during the day. Thus, early studies that reported a circadian decrement in TSH during the night actually revealed the inhibitory effect of sleep itself on TSH. In night-shift workers, without the inhibitory effect of sleep on TSH in the early night and with the circadian effects unmasked, TSH levels increase in the first half of the night.

The thyroid hormones themselves (tri-iodothyronine or T_3 and thyroxine or T_4) have been studied less with respect to circadian and sleep effects. However, conversely, the effect of thyroxine on sleep is well established. Hyperthyroid patients have motor hyperactivity, irritability and reduced sleep duration. Furthermore, insomnia, restless sleep and/or nightmares may be the presenting symptoms. Hypothyroid patients are frequently tired and somnolent, with increased amounts of total sleep time, although often with decreased sleep quality as a result of sleep-disordered breathing (obstructive sleep apnoea and/or alveolar hypoventilation, see Chapter 4).

Prolactin

Prolactin is also an anterior pituitary hormone. Its main established role is the initiation and maintenance of lactation.

Similar to GH and TSH, prolactin is affected primarily by sleep and only minimally by circadian regulation. In contrast to the inhibitory effect of sleep on TSH, sleep has a stimulatory effect on prolactin, even during daytime sleep (naps). In contrast to the sleep effect on GH, the sleep-related prolactin release sustains elevated prolactin levels throughout the night, rather than decreasing after the initial few hours of sleep, as is the case for the stimulatory effect of sleep on GH secretion. This difference may result from the specific SWS-related stimulatory effect of sleep on GH, whereas there are unknown relationships between prolactin secretion and specific sleep stages. In this way, sleep effects on prolactin resemble those of sleep effects on TSH, which remains inhibited during the entire sleep episode.

Thus, in the normal population (both men and women, in both follicular and luteal phases) the highest levels of prolactin are measured during sleep. It is unclear whether the effect of sleep is direct on prolactin secretion, mediated via TRH secretion (which results in increased serum levels of prolactin), or is mediated via a reduction in dopaminergic inhibition on prolactin production. In any case, the sleep dependence of the nocturnal rise in prolactin is evident from the much lower rises in nocturnal prolactin levels during sleep deprivation studies. In addition, under constant routine conditions, also in the absence of sleep, there is a small, but detectable, rise in prolactin levels in the habitual sleep time in the three groups studied (men and women in the follicular and luteal phases of the menstrual cycle). In women in their follicular phase, prolactin remains high throughout the night during constant routine conditions (similar to entrained conditions during sleep), whereas in those in the luteal phase under constant routine conditions prolactin levels fall after the initial rise and then rise again in the latter half of the night. In summary, prolactin levels are highest during the night, with sustained high levels throughout the night, primarily as a result of a stimulating effect of sleep, but also resulting from a circadian effect.

Gonadotrophins

Human pituitary gonadal function involves complex interactions between neural and endocrine influences. The anterior pituitary gland releases luteinizing hormone (LH) and follicle-stimulating hormone (FSH) in response to hypothalamic gonadotrophin-releasing hormone (GnRH), which is under the influence of central neurotransmitters and negative feedback by pituitary and gonadal hormones. LH and FSH influence the gonads to secrete testosterone (testes) and oestrogen and progesterone (ovaries). This complex system also depends on age (stage of development in children and menopause in women), sex and phase of the reproductive cycle in women. Initiation and maintenance of the reproductive axis depend on the pulsatile secretion of the hypothalamic GnRH. The pattern of GnRH secretion is constantly changing with age throughout development, from high levels during the neonatal period, through a period of quiescence in mid-childhood, followed by the sleep-entrained reactivation of the reproductive axis at the onset of puberty, and ultimately culminating in the adult pattern of pulsatile secretion, which in men is approximately every 2 hours and in women varies with the stage of the menstrual cycle.

Unlike other hormones, the effect of sleep on LH changes with factors such as developmental stage or sex. Sleep induces LH elevation in children, starting at approximately 2 years before the first clinical signs of puberty. At puberty, the amplitude of the nocturnal spikes markedly increases, although whether the reason is circadian or sleep itself is unresolved by previous studies. In pubertal children (both boys and girls), sleep augments LH secretion, with LH pulses measured mainly during NREM sleep. As a result, there is a tight relationship between the number of NREM/REM cycles and the number of LH pulses.

In adulthood, men continue to demonstrate sleep-related augmentation of LH secretion, primarily as a result of an increase in pulse amplitude and not of changes in pulse frequency. It is evident from the increase in LH pulse amplitudes during daytime naps that this sleep-related rise in LH secretion is primarily sleep effect rather than circadian influence. In contrast, adult women do not exhibit sleep-related augmentation of LH secretion and may even show some sleep-related inhibition of LH, especially in the follicular phase of the menstrual cycle. In contrast to the sleep effect on LH in adult men, in women this effect results primarily from a marked sleep-related decline in pulse frequency. There seems to be no effect of sleep on pulse frequency or pulse amplitude of LH in women in the luteal phase of the menstrual cycle.

In summary, the huge increase (almost 40-fold) in LH secretion from mid-childhood to sexual maturity results primarily from an amplification of a pre-existing ultradian rhythm of pulses, with a steadily increasing quantity of LH secreted per burst. The pulse frequency shows only a minimal increment from mid-childhood to the onset of puberty, with no further changes during puberty or adulthood. The duration of the secretory burst and the half-life of LH in the plasma remain largely unchanged from childhood to adulthood. Sleep-associated LH secretion begins in mid-childhood, enhances during puberty, continues in adult men, but is lost in adult women.

Although sleep affects gonadotrophic hormones, the gonadal hormones (androgens, oestrogen and progesterone) may influence sleep, mainly via their effect on breathing and potential sleep apnoea. These are discussed in Chapter 6.

Antidiuretic hormone

The posterior pituitary antidiuretic hormone (ADH, vasopressin) is a small peptide responsible for water reabsorption in the collecting ducts of the kidneys. The stimuli for ADH release are increased plasma osmolarity (perceived by osmoreceptors in the hypothalamus) and decreased blood volume (perceived by baroreceptors in the carotid sinus of the aortic arch). ADH secretion usually occurs at an osmolarity of more than 280, with an exponential rise with increasing osmolarity. However, even for a given osmolarity, ADH secretion increases during the night, which is believed to be a mechanism for preventing nocturia. Dysfunction of this nocturnal rise in ADH is believed to be one of the reasons for the persistence of nocturnal enuresis into adulthood (see Chapter 8). However, the role of ADH in nocturnal enuresis is controversial because some studies have reported failure of ADH to rise during the night (or ADH dysfunction during sleep), but others have reported a normal nocturnal rise of ADH in enuretic patients. Furthermore, only a minority of patients with diabetes insipidus (absence of ADH) suffers from nocturnal enuresis. Whether the nocturnal rise in ADH is a sleep or circadian effect is unknown because studies have not attempted to make this distinction.

Others

Both sleep and circadian rhythm play a role in the secretion and function of many other hormones as well, although these have been studied less than those mentioned above. Insulin secretion, for example, is primarily stimulated by glucose level. Therefore normally, as people do not eat during the night, glucose levels minimally decline, as do insulin levels. However, it has recently been shown that sleep inhibits the counter-regulatory hormone response to hypoglycaemia, and therefore children with type 1 diabetes mellitus (insulin dependent) are prone to develop nocturnal hypoglycaemia in response to over-treatment with insulin. Furthermore, we have recently reported that children with diabetes do not awaken with hypoglycaemia when it develops insidiously, and even respond with hypersynchronized slow-wave δ activity and deep sleep, exposing them to hypoglycaemia-related complications. In addition, sleep disruption can influence diabetes or even insulin sensitivity. Recent data suggest that sleep deprivation may result in insulin resistance.

There are also some data to suggest that sleep induces a rise in the levels of parathyroid hormone (PTH) and leptin, although these may be partially circadian effects, and more studies are needed to explore the exact role of sleep and circadian physiology on the secretion of these, as well as on other hormones.

chapter 3

Hypersomnia: an introduction

> Sleepy persons have a disposition to sleep on every occasion. They do so at all times, and in all places. They sleep after dinner; they sleep in the theater; they sleep in church. It is the same to them in what situation they may be placed: sleep is the great end of their existence – their occupation – their sole employment. Morpheus is the deity at whose shrine they worship – the only god whose inference over them is omnipotent.... Let them sail, or ride, or sit, or lie, or walk, sleep overtakes them; binds their faculties in torpor.... These are one dull, heavy-headed, drowsy mortals, whose sons and daughters of phlegm – with passion as inert as a clutch fog, and intellects as sluggish as the movements of the hypopotamus or leviathan.
>
> RD MacNish in *The Philosophy of Sleep*. NY: Appleton, 1830: 211–12.

A normal individual obtaining adequate sleep should be able to maintain wakefulness during the day with little to no difficulty. When such an individual consistently falls asleep unwillingly, this probably represents a clinical problem. The following outlines the definition, evaluation of severity and clinical approach to this situation.

Distinguishing sleepiness from fatigue

The first step in the approach to the complaint of daytime sleepiness is to distinguish between sleepiness and fatigue. Many people confuse the two, although these represent different clinical problems. Fatigue usually refers to a problem of lack of energy and/or exhaustion, but not necessarily sleepiness. Fatigue may be seen in a variety of medical and mental conditions, such as hypothyroidism, Addison's disease, anaemia, heart failure, rheumatic disorders, depression, chronic fatigue syndrome or any chronic illness condition. People with hypersomnolence, as opposed to fatigue, often fall asleep unintentionally. The tendency to fall asleep unintentionally can be quantified both subjectively and objectively.

Definition and quantification (subjective and objective)

Sleepiness reflects the tendency of an individual to fall asleep. Mild sleepiness describes the tendency to fall asleep unintentionally only during passive situations, when little attention is required. Moderate sleepiness describes unintentional sleep episodes during very mild physical activities which requires some degree of attention (e.g. driving or watching movies). Severe sleepiness expresses unintentional sleep episodes occurring during active situations such as eating or talking to someone.

Two widely accepted questionnaires measure subjective sleepiness. The Stanford Sleepiness Scale (SSS) represents the sleepiness at a given moment, and changes on a moment-by-moment basis according to the situation. The scale ranges between 1 and 7, and participants are asked to record the scale value of the statement that best describes their state of sleepiness (Table 12).

The SSS may be somewhat inaccurate in comparisons between people, but has been shown to be excellent in quantifying progressive steps in sleepiness in a given individual. It has been shown to be sensitive to sleep deprivation and diurnal variation in propensity to sleep, and to correlate negatively with performance. Thus, it is considered a good tool to measure sleepiness in an individual over time, but less valid in determining a chronic condition of somnolence and in between-person comparisons.

Table 12 The Stanford Sleepiness Scale (SSS)

1	Feeling active and vital, alert, wide awake
2	Functioning at high level, but not at peak, able to concentrate
3	Relaxed, awake, not at full alertness, responsive
4	A little foggy, not at peak, let down
5	Fogginess, beginning to lose interest in remaining awake, slowed down
6	Sleepiness, prefer to be lying down, fighting sleep, woozy
7	Almost in reverie, sleep onset soon, lost struggle to remain awake

The Epworth Sleepiness Scale (ESS) is another self-administered questionnaire (Table 13), which reflects the person's general level of daytime sleepiness. In its initial introduction in 1991, it had been shown to correlate with objective measurements of sleepiness (the MSLT, see below) and with sleep-disordered breathing severity in sleep apnoea patients. Furthermore, it negatively correlated with the minimum oxygen saturation in patients with sleep apnoea, and did not differ between simple snorers and controls. It was designed to measure and quantify sleep propensity rather than fatigue, as manifested by the tendency to fall asleep in a variety of conditions:

The numbers selected in Table 13 for the eight situations are added together to give a score for each person between 0 and 24. The higher the score, the sleepier the patient, generally with scores up to 6–7 considered normal, 8–12 mild sleepiness, 13–17 moderate sleepiness, and 18 and above severe sleepiness. As stated, the ESS reflects a general level of sleepiness. It is considered to be independent of short-term variations in sleepiness and the time of the day, and is consistent from day to day. It has been shown to be consistently higher in conditions associated with daytime somnolence (such as sleep apnoea, narcolepsy, idiopathic hypersomnolence), and normal in other sleep disturbances such as insomnia. However, again it reflects subjective assessment of sleepiness, without objective documentation.

For objective measurement of sleepiness, the Multiple Sleep Latency Test (MSLT) has been developed, with the working hypothesis that the

Table 13 The Epworth Sleepiness Scale (ESS)

How likely are you to doze off or fall asleep in the following situations, in contrast to feeling just tired? This refers to your usual way of life in recent times. Even if you have not done some of these things recently, try to work out how they would have affected you. Use the following scale to choose the most appropriate number for each situation:

0 = would never doze
1 = slight chance of dozing
2 = moderate chance of dozing
3 = high chance of dozing

Situation	*Score*	*0*	*1*	*2*	*3*
Sitting and reading					
Watching TV					
Sitting inactive in a public place (theatre, meeting)					
As a passenger in a car for an hour without a break					
Lying down to rest in the afternoon when circumstances permit					
Sitting and talking to someone					
Sitting quietly after lunch without alcohol					
In a car, while stopped for a few minutes in the traffic					
Total					

drowsier the person, the more rapidly he or she should fall asleep under favourable conditions. The MSLT should be conducted after a nocturnal polysomnographic recording to ensure an undisturbed preceding night's sleep. Ideally, the patient should complete a sleep diary for 1–2 weeks before the study because the MSLT may be influenced by sleep for up to 7 nights beforehand. As therapy for many causes of hypersomnia requires stimulants (with potential for abuse), a urine drug screen on the morning of the MSLT is also encouraged. Then, five sleep latency tests are performed in a quiet and dark room at 2-hour intervals, beginning 1.5–3 hours after the end of the nocturnal recording. On each occasion, the patient is encouraged to fall asleep, and is given 20 min to do so. If a patient does not fall asleep in 20 min, that specific opportunity is terminated, and the patient is asked to get out of bed and avoid sleeping. If a patient falls asleep on every given occasion, the test continues for an additional 15 min unless rapid eye movement (REM) sleep occurs. If unequivocal REM sleep occurs, the test is terminated. In each test, sleep latency is determined as the time elapsed between lights out and sleep onset. REM latency is taken as the time between sleep onset and REM onset. If, in a given test, the patient did not fall asleep, that specific test is considered as a sleep latency of 20 min. A single summary value for sleep latency is calculated as the average sleep latency across the five tests. A mean MSLT of 10–15 min is considered mild sleepiness, 5–10 min is considered moderate sleepiness, and less than 5 min reflects severe sleepiness. These values are summarized in Table 14.

Consequences (behavioural and functional)

Hypersomnolence results in several consequences, some of which resemble those of sleep deprivation (see Table 7). As a direct consequence of sleepiness, affected individuals are vulnerable to sleep-related accidents (road and work accidents). They also tend to fall asleep in undesired and embarrassing situations, and may therefore be prone to social maladjustment and decreased marital satisfaction. Sometimes the behavioural manifestation of sleepiness is, paradoxically, hyperactivity, especially in children. Other behavioural and mood manifestations of sleepiness may include irritability, nervousness, violence, depression and low self-

Table 14 Quantitative evaluation of subjective and objective sleepiness

Sleepiness	*MSLT (min)*	*ESS*
Mild	11–15	8–12
Moderate	6–10	13–17
Severe	≤5	≥18

MSLT, Multiple Sleep Latency Test; ESS, Epworth Sleepiness Scale.

esteem. Functional and cognitive impairment are also characteristic of all conditions associated with daytime sleepiness. Children suffer from low school achievement, and adults from decreased academic and occupational performance. Thus, daytime somnolence is a serious condition that requires investigation, diagnosis and treatment.

chapter 4

Sleep apnoea syndrome

Sleep of an Obese Poulterer

When in sound sleep a very peculiar state of the glottis is observed, a spasmodic closure entirely suspending respiration. The thorax and abdomen are seen to heave from fruitless contractions of the inspiratory and expiratory muscles; their efforts increase in violence for about a minute or a minute and a half, the skin meantime becoming more and more cyanosed, until at last, when the condition to the onlooker is most alarming, the glottic obstruction yields, a series of long inspirations and expirations follows, and cyanosis disappears. This acute dyspnoeic attack does not awaken the patient. . . . If in the midst of the dyspnoeic attack he is forcibly aroused, the glottic spasm at once relaxes. The night nurses state that these attacks go on throughout the night.

Richard Caton. *Clin Soc Tran* 1889; 22: 133–7.

The sleep apnoea syndrome is characterized by frequent cessations of breathing during sleep. It is usually associated with excessive daytime sleepiness. However, in some cases (mainly central sleep apnoea) it may be associated with insomnia. Cessation of breathing during sleep can be partial (decreased tidal volume, hypopnoea) or complete (apnoea), which may result from obstruction of the upper airway (obstructive apnoea), loss of ventilatory effort (central apnoea) or a combination of the two (mixed apnoea). The type of event determines the diagnosis of central or obstructive sleep apnoea.

When most of the events are obstructive or mixed, obstructive sleep apnoea (OSA) is diagnosed, whereas for a diagnosis of pure central sleep apnoea (CSA) at least 80% of the events are required to be of central origin (see later). When most of the events are mixed, it is usually diagnosed as OSA. The severity of the syndrome, in both OSA and CSA, is primarily determined by the rate of sleep-disordered breathing events per hour of sleep (RDI or respiratory disturbance index; AHI or apnoea–hypopnoea index) and the magnitude of associated oxygen desaturations. As both hypopnoeas and complete apnoeas result in arousals from sleep, the distinction between them is not considered important from a severity point of view.

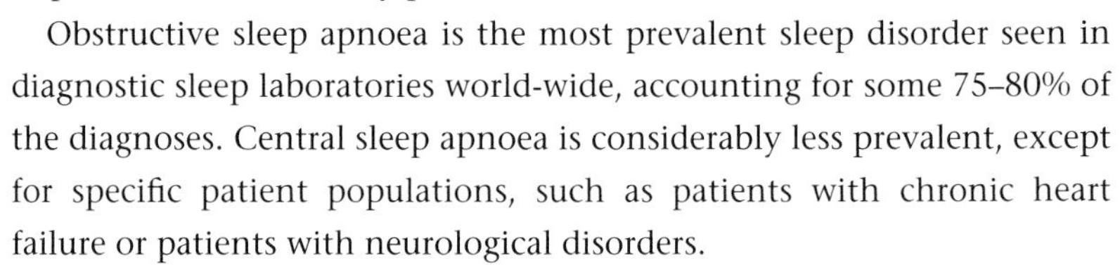

Obstructive sleep apnoea is the most prevalent sleep disorder seen in diagnostic sleep laboratories world-wide, accounting for some 75–80% of the diagnoses. Central sleep apnoea is considerably less prevalent, except for specific patient populations, such as patients with chronic heart failure or patients with neurological disorders.

Obstructive sleep apnoea

Definition and epidemiology

Obstructive apnoea is defined as the cessation of airflow despite continuing respiratory effort (Figure 5). When such events are seen repetitively, then OSA is diagnosed. This is a very common disorder. In a large population-based study the prevalence of sleep-disordered breathing (RDI > 5 events per hour) was found to be 9% in women and 24% in men. In elderly people, the prevalence of sleep-disordered breathing is much higher, with an estimated prevalence of 80% for an RDI of >5. A finding of RDI > 5 is insufficient for a diagnosis of OSA; it should be accompanied by characteristic complaints, most notably daytime somnolence. Using this definition, a prevalence of 2% in middle-aged women and 4% in middle-aged men has been reported. This increases to up to 30% in

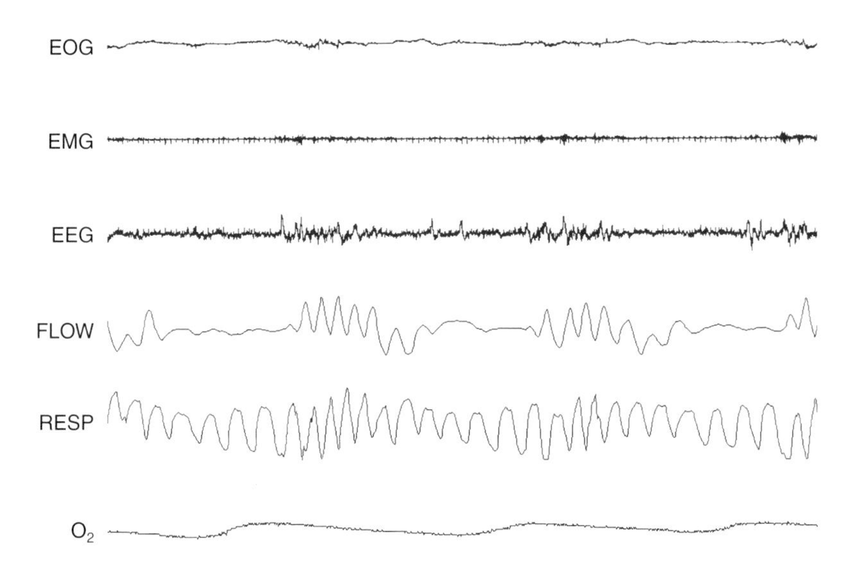

Figure 5 *An example of obstructive sleep apnoeas (2 min). EOG, electrooculogram; EMG, electromyogram; EEG, electroencephalogram; Flow, airflow; RESP, respiratory effort; and O_2, oxygen saturation.*

elderly people. It should be noted, however, that, although subjective sleepiness is currently required for the diagnosis of OSA, there are data to suggest that people may be unaware of their sleepiness, and that important complications of obstructive apnoea may occur in the absence of sleepiness (e.g. hypertension). Thus, the prevalence of OSA could be higher if cardiovascular complications were included in the definition. Table 15 presents the RDIs and oxygen saturation values representing different severity levels of the syndrome.

Table 15 Severity indices of obstructive sleep apnoea

	RDI (events/h)	*Minimum O_2 saturation (%)*
Normal	<5	>95
Mild	5–19	>85
Moderate	20–39	>65
Severe	>40	<65

History and physical examination

Snoring, witnessed apnoeic episodes, daytime fatigue/sleepiness, choking and/or gasping during sleep are the most common complaints of OSA patients. Additional symptoms include impaired concentration/ cognitive abilities (e.g. memory impairment), morning headaches plus dry mouth, and possibly also depression and sexual impotence. In children, daytime hypersomnolence is less common than in adults, but, on the other hand, many parents report daytime hyperactivity, attention deficit and mouth-breathing while children are awake (caused by enlargement of the adenoids) and frequent upper respiratory infections.

The physical examination adds little to the diagnosis, but it can raise suspicion, especially in children, in whom it is very common to find hypertrophy of the adenoids and tonsils. In adults the examination may show obesity, an increased neck circumference, a small, crowded posterior pharyngeal space (with or without enlarged tonsils), nasal obstruction, lower extremity oedema and/or systemic hypertension. Based just on history and physical examination, the ability to predict OSA is fairly poor.

Diagnosis

The gold standard for the diagnosis of OSA is in-laboratory full-night polysomnography (PSG). Ideally 6 hours of sleep are recorded, including all sleep positions and all sleep stages. By counting all respiratory disturbance events and dividing them by the total number of hours of sleep, the RDI is determined. Some laboratories perform 'split-night' studies (i.e. diagnose OSA in the first half of the night, and adjust CPAP (continuous positive airway pressure) treatment (see later) during the second half, if there is a finding of an RDI > 20/h in the first half. Although it virtually reduces the cost, this method may be less accurate in the diagnosis as a result of the relatively short sleep time with the potential lack of REM sleep or supine sleep in the diagnostic half. Home monitoring has also been suggested for the diagnosis of OSA. Ambulatory devices have initially included oximetry alone, but other methods of home monitoring, including a variety of recorded channels such as breathing effort and airflow, body movements and peripheral arterial tone, are also used.

Risk factors

Anatomy

The most recognized risk factor for OSA is anatomical narrowing of the upper airway. Studies using a variety of imaging techniques (computed tomography [CT], magnetic resonance imaging [MRI]), acoustic reflection, cephalometrics) have demonstrated a small pharyngeal airway in patients with apnoea, with the smallest airway luminal size generally occurring at the level of the velopharynx. Narrowing of the upper airways can result from obesity (see later), or from specific craniofacial abnormalities such as retrognathia, micrognathia (e.g. Pierre–Robin sequence), midface hypoplasia (e.g. Down's, Crouzon's and Apert's syndromes, and achondroplasia), mandibular hypoplasia (e.g. Cornelia De Lange syndrome), increased soft tissue size such as macroglossia (e.g. Down's syndrome or acromegaly), hypertrophy of the tonsils and adenoids (which are especially important in children), or increased uvula size or long soft palate.

Although the most common site of obstruction is the retropalatal or retroglossal region (see Figure 6), nasal anatomy also plays a role in OSA. Increased nasal resistance can result in increased negative suction pressure by the diaphragm, and increased tendency of the upper airways to collapse. Thus, nasal polyps, a deflected nasal septum or chronic nasal congestion also contribute to OSA. Most importantly, measurement of the critical pressure (P_{crit}), which is needed to close (completely collapse) the upper airway of sleep apnoea patients undergoing general anaesthesia, revealed a positive P_{crit}, in comparison to negative values in normal controls. Under these conditions of complete neuromuscular paralysis, only anatomical factors are important in pharyngeal patency. Thus, in sleep apnoea patients, the airway was collapsed at atmospheric pressure and required positive pressure to reopen. Normal controls, on the other hand, had patent airways at atmospheric pressure and required suction (negative pressure) to collapse the pharynx.

Obesity

Obesity is an important risk factor for the development of OSA. Most OSA patients are overweight, and OSA is substantially more common in

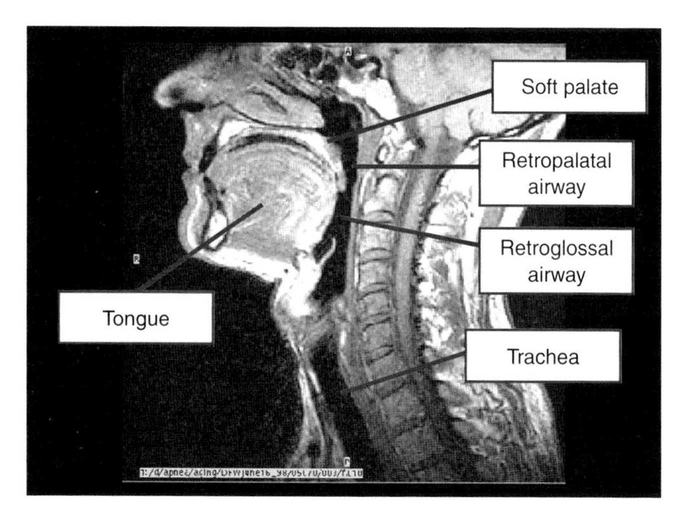

Figure 6 *Magnetic resonance image of a normal subject. A mid-sagittal section of a normal individual illustrating the relevant anatomy. Collapse in obstructive sleep apnoea patients tends to occur behind the palate and/or tongue (retropalatal/retroglossal).*

obese individuals. In morbidly obese patients (body mass index or BMI of 40 kg/m^2 or more), at least 70% suffer from OSA. The odds ratio of sleep apnoea in obese versus non-obese people has been reported to be between 8 and 14. The exact mechanism(s) by which obesity causes OSA is unclear. It probably relates to a combination of several mechanisms such as upper airway narrowing (as stated above), weakening of upper airway muscles, decreasing lung volumes, etc. Central obesity is considered more relevant for OSA than general obesity, and this may be one of the reasons for the sex-related differences in OSA (see below). Neck circumference index and waist–hip ratio (WHR) have been recognized as better predictors of OSA than obesity in general. Fat deposits in the neck may result in upper airway luminal narrowing and muscle weakening. Additional evidence for the close association between obesity and OSA can be concluded from the fact that massive weight reduction in morbidly obese OSA patients results in many cases, in complete cure of the syndrome. Obesity also plays a role in children's OSA, although to a lesser extent than in adults. (See Figure 7.)

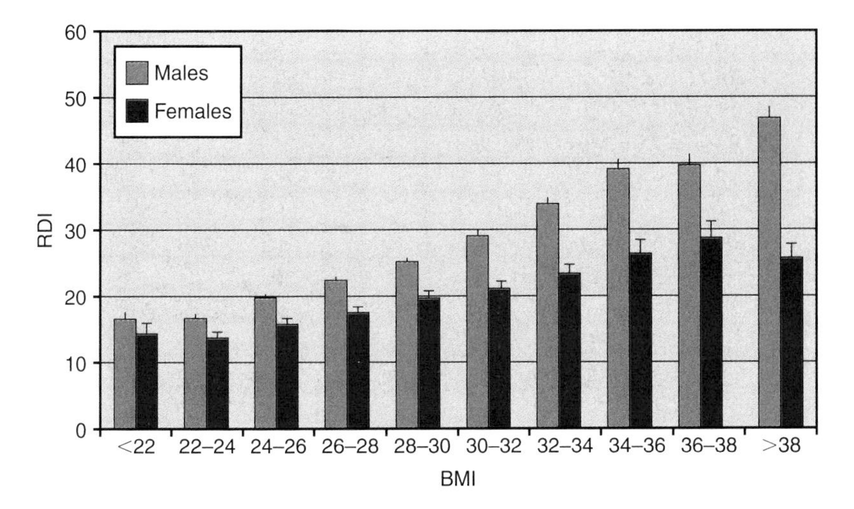

Figure 7 *Relationship between BMI and RDI in sleep apnoea. Data for 5000 men and 1000 women studied in the Technion Sleep Disorders Centre are presented.*

Age

It is well documented that OSA is age dependent (see also Figure 8). There is a progressive increase in the prevalence of OSA, at least up to the sixth or seventh decade of life, independent of BMI. The mechanism is unclear, because no obvious anatomical or physiological factors that predispose to an increased risk of apnoea have been found with ageing. The prevalence of OSA is relatively high in small children (ages 3–5), because they tend to have narrow airways as a result of enlargement of the adenoids and tonsils. Then, it decreases dramatically in adolescents and young adults, and increases in middle-aged and elderly people. Longitudinal studies in OSA patients have failed, however, to demonstrate clear-cut worsening over time (there are conflicting reports in this regard), and the natural history of OSA is unclear at this time. Thus, sleep apnoea may progress with time if weight is gained, but may remain steady if there are no additional risk factors.

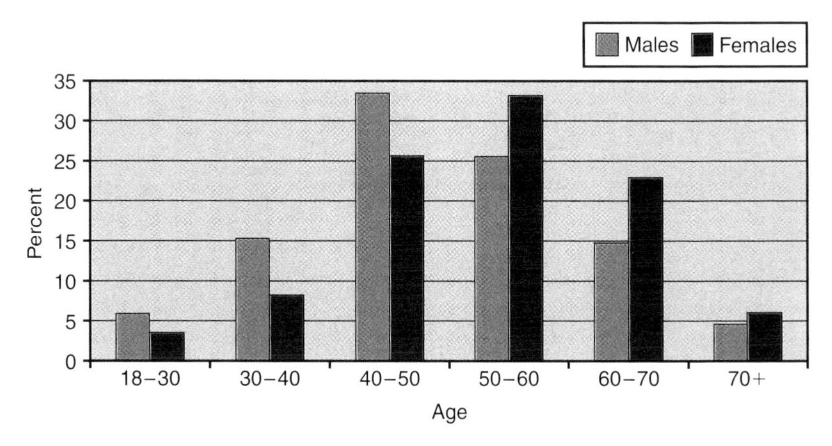

Figure 8 *Age distribution of 5000 men and 1000 women with obstructive sleep apnoea syndrome, studied at the Technion Sleep Disorders Centre. Note that the women with sleep apnoea tend to be older than the men.*

Sex

Male sex is an important risk factor for the development of OSA. In population-based studies men have been found to have between a two- and fivefold increased risk of OSA compared with weight-matched women. In sleep clinic populations, the men/women ratio is even higher, up to 8–10. The reasons for this sex difference are not clear. Several explanations have been proposed such as sex-related differences in anatomy and physiology of the upper airway and in respiratory control system, and the possibility that androgens may inhibit upper airway muscle activity in men, whereas oestrogen and progesterone may stimulate respiration in women. Also, central obesity in men may compromise their airways compared with the peripherally-distributed fat in women, and other genetic sex-related anatomical differences in the upper airway (also possibly hormone mediated) may play a role.

The findings that the prevalence of OSA in women increases postmenopausally, and that oestrogen plus progesterone replacement therapy in postmenopausal women increases upper airway muscle activation and decreases OSA, support the role of these hormones. However, hormonal therapy for men failed to abolish OSA, which indicates that hormonal differences alone cannot explain the sex-related differences in

OSA. In children there are no sex-related differences in OSA, which suggests that these differences develop over time or that the pathophysiology of OSA differs between children and adults.

Genetics

There is evidence that genetic factors are important in OSA, although their exact role is unclear. Sleep-disordered breathing clusters together in families, and OSA is substantially more prevalent in offspring of OSA patients. The relative risk of OSA may be two- to fourfold greater in first-degree relatives. Genetic factors may explain as much as 40% of the variance in RDI. The familial factors remain significant after adjustment for BMI and cephalometric measurements. Moreover, unaffected offspring of OSA patients are more vulnerable to provocative tests than controls. They have been shown to respond with increased upper airway collapse in response to inspiratory resistive loading. Several case reports of families have suggested an autosomal dominant pattern of inheritance, but at this time it is more likely that inheritance is multifactorial. Interestingly, one study not only found an increased risk for sleep apnoea in lean relatives of OSA subjects, but also a higher incidence of the sudden infant death syndrome (SIDS) in these families as well.

Other risk factors

Several additional specific risk factors are known for OSA. These include some diseases such as hypothyroidism (mainly caused by myxoedema and decreased upper airway muscle function) and acromegaly (mainly resulting from macroglossia and potentially disordered ventilatory control stability). Cerebrovascular accidents and brain-stem lesions may result in obstructive apnoeas, although in these cases central apnoeas are more common. Neuromuscular diseases are also predisposing factors, which can result in hypoventilation and sleep-disordered breathing events of both central and obstructive types (see the CSA section). These include muscular dystrophies such as Duchenne and myotonic dystrophies, myopathies such as Nemaline-Rod myopathy or acid-maltase deficiency, and neuropathies such as Charcot–Marie–Tooth peripheral neuropathy or the post-polio syndrome.

Table 16 Risk factors for obstructive sleep apnoea

Risk factor	*Comments*
Upper airway anatomy	Retrognathia, micrognathia, macroglossia, hypertrophy of tonsils or adenoids, increased uvula size, long soft palate, nasal narrowing
Obesity	Increases, especially with central obesity
Age and sex	OSA is more prevalent in men, and the prevalence increases with age
Endocrine	Hypothyroidism, acromegaly
Genetic	OSA clusters in families, with a relative risk of two- to fourfold in first-degree relatives
Neuromuscular	Myopathies, muscular dystrophies, neuropathies
Extrinsic	Alcohol, CNS depressants (hypnotics, opioids)

In addition, there is an increased risk of having apnoeas after the use of CNS depressants such as hypnotics, opioids or alcohol.

Chronic lung disease does not pose a direct risk factor for OSA, but in both obstructive and restrictive lung disease OSA tends to be more severe, with deeper events of oxygen desaturation, resulting from hypoventilation and the low lung reserve. In addition, some abnormalities are common risk factors for both lung disease and OSA, such as obesity, kyphoscoliosis and neuromuscular diseases. Table 16 summarizes the risk factors for OSA.

Pathophysiology

Although all the above-mentioned risk factors exist during both wakefulness and sleep, apnoeas exist only in sleep, yielding an additional factor, presumably functional, that is present exclusively during sleep and allows apnoea to occur. This factor seems to be the loss of upper airway muscle activation. During wakefulness, airway patency can be maintained by increased neural activation of pharyngeal dilator muscles, such as the genioglossus, tensor palatini, geniohyoid and sternohyoid. However, at sleep onset, muscle activity falls, allowing upper airway collapse, most commonly at the level of the soft palate.

Some speculate that the evolution of speech in humans, which demanded substantial laryngeal motility, led to the loss of rigid support of the hyoid bone, which is anchored to the styloid process of the skull in most mammals. This rendered the pharyngeal airway of humans largely dependent on soft tissue and dilator muscle activation to maintain patency. The portion of the upper airway most vulnerable to collapse lies between the choanae (back of the nose) and the epiglottis. During wakefulness, pharyngeal dilator muscles are generally able to maintain patency in this portion of the airway, independent of anatomical factors. However, the extent to which the airway is dependent on muscle activation is quite variable. An individual with an anatomically large airway may have a minimal requirement for pharyngeal muscle activity, whereas a patient with a small one may be critically dependent on dilator function to maintain patency. As a result of insufficient muscle activation, at the onset of inspiration, when luminal pressure becomes subatmospheric (i.e. negative), the upper airways collapse.

Pharyngeal dilator muscle activity therefore must increase to maintain patency, and this increase must occur before the initiation of inspiration. During expiration the luminal pressure becomes positive, thereby supporting the airway even in the absence of phasic muscle activity.

It is not very well understood why dilator muscles lose their activity during sleep. The primary stimuli responsible for these muscles' activation are central activation, as part of the respiratory sequence, and a local reflex mechanism responding to negative pressure. Upper airway muscle activation normally occurs 50–150 ms before inspiratory airflow on each breath (i.e. 'pre-activation'), thus anticipating the negative pressure generated by the diaphragm. Losing this delicately orchestrated time sequence may result in obstructive apnoeas.

The primary stimulus for the local reflex activation of the upper airway muscle is negative pressure, although CO_2 may play a role (during wakefulness) as well. During sleep, there is a marked attenuation or loss of this locally mediated reflex activation even in normal individuals. Thus, an anatomically small airway that is dependent on reflex-driven dilator muscle activity to maintain patency will be vulnerable to collapse during sleep.

Consequences

The physiological consequences of apnoea are a rise in the arterial CO_2 partial pressure ($Paco_2$), a fall in Pao_2 and increasing ventilatory effort against an occluded airway. As apnoea progresses, both systemic and pulmonary artery pressures rise, reaching a peak immediately after the termination of the apnoea. Left and right ventricular output falls at this point, and the activity of the sympathetic nervous system increases markedly, leading to increased vascular resistance. This transient arousal from sleep re-establishes the airway and ventilation. The individual subsequently returns to sleep and the cycle begins again, to be repeated frequently over the course of the night. The clinical consequences seen in OSA patients probably occur as a result of one or more of these factors.

The major clinical consequences of OSA are summarized in Table 17.

Neurocognitive effects

Excessive daytime sleepiness (EDS) is the most common presenting complaint of patients with OSA, being reported in up to 90% of such patients. The mechanism is probably sleep fragmentation, because other causes of sleep disruption and even experimental sleep fragmentation may result in EDS. Although there is a general tendency for severe OSA patients to be sleepier than patients with mild or moderate OSA, there is only a poor correlation between subjective (Epworth Sleepiness Scale or

Table 17 Consequences of obstructive sleep apnoea

Neurocognitive	Excessive daytime sleepiness, decreased cognitive performance, increased road traffic and work accidents, depression?
Cardiovascular	Systemic and pulmonary hypertension, coronary artery disease, congestive heart failure, arrhythmias, CVA
Social	Decreased quality of life, poor sexual function, partner's sleep disorders, increased divorce rate
Mortality	Increased risk in young and middle age

CVA, cerebrovascular accident.

ESS) or objective (Multiple Sleep Latency Test or MSLT) measures of sleepiness and sleep apnoea indices. This may result from a less than ideal assessment of arousals from sleep. Some recent studies assessing subcortical (autonomic) arousals resulted in improvement of the relationship between sleep disruption indices and sleepiness. Successful treatment of OSA results in improvement of both subjective and objective sleepiness.

An increased rate of accidents (both road traffic and at work) in OSA is well documented, and probably can also be attributed to the increased daytime somnolence, although some impaired cognitive function (e.g. judgement) may also play a role. Cognitive performance is clearly impaired in patients with sleep apnoea. This may be manifested as deterioration of memory, intellectual capacity and motor coordination. The ability to perform psychomotor vigilance tasks such as visual reaction, and auditory learning was also shown to be impaired in sleep apnoea. The mechanism by which OSA results in cognitive impairment is probably multifactorial, potentially resulting from the effects of chronic sleep deprivation and recurrent hypoxaemia. Several studies have found increased prevalence of depression in OSA, although there is no consensus on this finding.

Accounts of a sleepy physician

I began the study of medicine, and it was during the lectures' hours that I was first troubled with my inability to keep awake. During the three years of my attendance upon medical lectures I do not think there was a single day when I did not at least once during the lectures either go soundly asleep or pass into a state of semi-unconsciousness. . . .

This condition of things has grown steadily worse, until now I seldom can read more than half an hour – often not longer than fifteen minutes – without falling asleep. I would often, thinking it might be only a mental habit which could be broken by opposition, fight against this sleepiness for hours. . . . I have gone

> to sleep while making a vaginal examination in case of labour. Three times during the writing of a single prescription I have nodded off in a momentary doze. I have gone to sleep in a dental chair while the pounding of gold filling was going on.
>
> From the Minutes of the NY Neurological Society, 3 June 1884: 617.

Cardiovascular consequences

Probably the most important adverse effects of OSA, which may result in increased mortality, are in the cardiovascular system. Systemic hypertension is the best documented and studied consequence of OSA, with both epidemiological and experimental data to support it.

There is compelling evidence that sleep apnoea is associated with and contributes to systemic hypertension, potentially in a dose–response fashion. Blood pressure and percentage hypertension were reported to increase linearly with the increase in the severity of sleep apnoea, as indicated by the RDI. The RDI was a significant predictor of both systolic and diastolic blood pressure after adjustment for age, BMI and sex. The relative contribution of RDI to blood pressure was more important than that of BMI. Based on blood pressure measurements obtained from a large cohort of sleep apnoea patients, it was found that each additional apnoeic episode per hour of sleep increases the odds of having hypertension by approximately 1%, whereas a 10% decrease in nocturnal oxygen saturation increases the odds by 13% (Figure 9). More recently, a 10-year follow-up of a population-based study of 2668 middle-aged men reported that 12.5% of habitual snorers developed hypertension compared with only 7.4% of non-snoring men. Habitual snoring was found to be an independent predictor for the development of hypertension after controlling for age, BMI, smoking, alcohol use and exercise level.

The causal relationship between sleep apnoea and systemic hypertension was also supported in a study employing an animal model. By experimentally generating OSA in dogs, investigators from Toronto showed that repeated apnoeas were associated with substantial increases

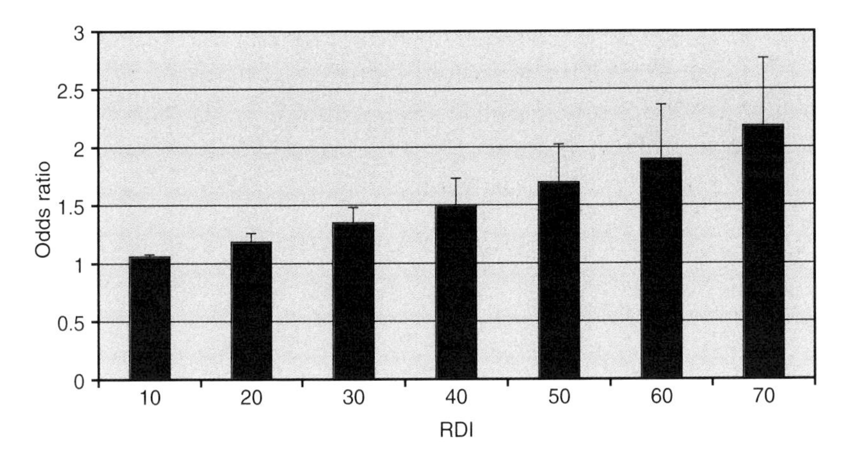

Figure 9 *Risk of hypertension in patients with increasing severity of sleep apnoea as indexed by RDI in comparison with people with RDI < 5. Data modified from Lavie, Herer and Hoffstein (*BMJ *2000).*

in both nocturnal and daytime blood pressure within about 4 weeks. Recurrent auditory arousals without airway obstruction were associated with nocturnal blood pressure elevation but not with sustained daytime hypertension. This suggests that recurrent arousals do not, by themselves, lead to sustained hypertension, thus suggesting a more prominent role for the recurrent hypoxaemia than the sympathetic activation alone. In addition, several studies have shown that treatment of sleep apnoea may lead to a reduction in blood pressure.

The picture is less clear with respect to pulmonary hypertension. Early reports have shown increased pulmonary hypertension in OSA patients, probably as a result of the recurrent hypoxaemia and hypercapnia. This was associated with decreased right heart function, including right heart failure and cor pulmonale. However, several more recent studies have found that OSA alone is not sufficient for the development of substantial pulmonary hypertension, and probably a daytime abnormality in arterial blood gases is necessary as well. Thus, severe pulmonary hypertension from OSA is generally seen only with daytime hypercapnia (e.g. obesity hypoventilation syndrome) or a pulmonary parenchymal abnormality (e.g. emphysema).

In children, however, data show that severe sleep apnoea results in decreased right ventricular ejection fraction, right ventricular hypertrophy and, if untreated, right heart failure.

There are some data to support an association between sleep apnoea and coronary artery disease (CAD), although this association is less clear than with hypertension. Patients with both CAD and OSA have been shown to suffer from nocturnal ischaemic events during sleep, and effective treatment of the OSA ameliorates the nocturnal ischaemia. In addition, the prevalence of OSA is higher in patients with CAD than in controls. Some reports associated sleep apnoea with congestive heart disease, although it is not always clear which was the cause and which the result (see Central sleep apnoea). Stroke may similarly be a cause or effect of OSA. Some data demonstrated that snoring and apnoea increased the risk for a cerebrovascular accident (CVA), and some data showed increased prevalence of apnoea status post stroke.

The mechanism for both CAD and CVA as a result of OSA may be speculated to be endothelial dysfunction in OSA leading to atherosclerosis, as was indeed recently evident from the decreased nitric oxide production in these patients, and an increase in the rate of biochemical markers of atherosclerosis.

Several arrhythmias have been reported in OSA. The most common one appears to be bradycardia, with extremes of sinus pauses of up to 10 s. Other arrhythmias include ventricular premature beats (VPBs), premature ventricular contractions (PVCs) and even ventricular tachycardia. There are some data showing that these arrhythmias improved with apnoea therapy.

Social consequences

As a result of the combination of daytime somnolence, decreased cognitive function, potential impotence in men, potential gastro-oesophageal reflex and heartburn, headaches and decreased self-esteem, measures of quality of life clearly deteriorate with sleep-disordered breathing. Patients with apnoea generally report diminished functional level and satisfaction on general scales such as the SF-36, with lower social function, decreased libido, poor sexual function, poor adjustment and a decreased sense of mental health and energy. All seem to improve with treatment. The loud snoring as well as fear about stopping breathing result in decreased quality of sleep in the partners of sleep apnoea patients. This may lead to increased irritability (see Chapter 7), and some studies even reported increased divorce rate in families if one partner suffered from sleep apnoea.

Mortality

Obstructive sleep apnoea was reported to be an independent risk factor for mortality, in young and middle-aged patients. In a retrospective review of 385 male patients with sleep apnoea, one study found that an apnoea index (AI) of more than 20/h was associated with a significantly reduced survival at 8 years compared with those with an AI < 20. This reduced survival was not observed in treated patients or in patients older than 50 years. Likewise, based on the data obtained from 1600 OSA patients, we found increased mortality from cardiovascular and respiratory causes only in patients younger than 50 years. Recently, we replicated these findings with a considerably larger cohort of 28 000 patients. Similar findings were reported from Sweden in a 10-year follow-up study of individuals who complained of snoring and EDS. These findings suggest a possible adaptation of the cardiovascular mechanisms to the nightly insults.

Treatment

Current therapeutic strategies for OSA are aimed at either enlarging the pharyngeal airway and thereby rendering it less susceptible to collapse, or using positive airway pressure to splint the airway pneumatically during sleep (Table 18).

Behavioural therapy

All patients with OSA should be given advice about the avoidance of activities or agents that may worsen their disease. These include alcohol consumption before sleep, use of sedatives/hypnotics (benzodiazapines, opioids, zolpidem) and sleep deprivation.

Table 18 Treatment options of obstructive sleep apnoea

Treatment	*Comments*
Behavioural	Avoidance of alcohol and CNS depressants, weight reduction, positional therapy
Surgical	Nasal surgery, somnoplasty, LAUP, UPPP, genioglossal advancement with hyoid myotomy, MMA, tracheostomy
Mechanical	Oral appliances, CPAP
Pharmacological	Nasal decongestants, oxygen, medroxyprogesterone, protriptyline, others

CPAP,continuous positive airway pressure; LAUP, laser-assisted uvuloplasty; MMA, maxillomandibular advancement; UPPP, uvulopalatopharynoplasty.

Weight reduction

As obesity is the single most important predictor of apnoea, weight loss would be expected to lead to an increase in upper airway dimensions and an improvement in sleep-disordered breathing. Indeed, it has been shown that weight loss can lead to a decrease in the RDI, reduced BP, improved sleep efficiency, decreased snoring and improved oxygenation. The most dramatic results have been reported with surgical weight loss, although on long-term follow-up of patients undergoing gastric reduction surgery, a recurrence of substantial apnoea has been observed in some, despite only minimal weight gain. It should be recognized, however, that substantial weight loss by non-surgical means is both difficult to achieve and even harder to sustain. Therefore, weight loss is an effective but difficult long-term therapeutic strategy. In addition, it usually improves, although it does not totally abolish, the apnoea.

Positional therapy

In most patients, apnoea is considerably worse in the supine posture, with some patients having apnoeas only in that position. Studies have shown that upper airway dimensions, airflow resistance and airway collapsibility all deteriorate in the supine posture, explaining this positional effect. For such patients behavioural techniques aimed at keeping the patient in the lateral decubitus position during sleep may offer some benefit. This has been accomplished by sewing an uncomfortable object into the back of the nightshirt or positional alarms. Unfortunately, patients acceptance of this therapy is suboptimal, with an important benefit likely only for those with relatively mild apnoea.

Continuous positive airway pressure

Since its initial description in 1981, continuous positive airway pressure (CPAP), applied via a nasal mask, has been the primary therapy for patients with OSA. CPAP effectively eliminates velopharyngeal collapse essentially in all individuals who use it. The prescribed CPAP pressure is typically determined in the sleep laboratory, taking into consideration all sleep stages and all body positions. There is strong evidence supporting improvements with nasal CPAP on all measures of apnoea, including breathing during sleep, daytime alertness, neurocognitive functions, mood, and even cardiovascular sequelae.

Despite CPAP's almost universal effectiveness in treating sleep apnoea, it still suffers from major compliance limitations. First, only about two-thirds of patients who are offered CPAP are willing to use it. Second, estimates from various studies suggest that, on average, patients only use the treatment 4–5 hours per night.

To improve patient adherence, several strategies have been employed: first, patient habituation to the mask before actually using the therapy may be helpful. This can help to provide an optimal fit, and alleviate the initial discomfort and anxiety associated with the use of the CPAP mask. It also allows the opportunity to change the type of mask or the type of strap according to patient comfort. Issues such as mouth leak, which can lead to morning mouth dryness, can be improved with the use of a chin strap attached to the nasal mask apparatus.

Second, benzodiazepines have been used initially to alleviate anxiety associated with CPAP therapy. In certain patients, a short course of anxiolytics, or hypnotics, may improve patient acceptance of this treatment and allow the onset of sleep. The potentially deleterious effect of these medications on untreated apnoea makes their use undesirable if the apnoea remains untreated.

Third, nasal symptomatology includes drying and congestion which is amenable to treatment with heated humidification of the inspired air. This is because nasal congestion is a manifestation of the body's attempt to humidify the incoming air if inadequate moisture is detected. Other causes of nasal congestion and rhinitis, such as seasonal allergic rhinitis and vasomotor rhinitis, often respond to treatments with anticholinergic nasal sprays, intranasal steroids and immunotherapy.

Fourth, excessive air pressure is an occasional complaint of CPAP users. This is caused partly by the need to exhale against positive pressure, which can slightly increase the effort and discomfort associated with breathing. One strategy to reduce this symptom is bi-level positive airway pressure (BIPAP), which allows the clinician to prescribe different levels of pressure for inspiration and expiration. The routine use of BIPAP therapy has not been shown to improve patient adherence; however, occasional patients with a high CPAP pressure requirement, who specifically complain about the air pressure, may be better served by this treatment. In addition, individuals with the pickwickian syndrome (with daytime alveolar hypoventilation resulting in hypercapnia), in combination with OSA, may benefit from BIPAP to improve nocturnal ventilation.

Similarly, auto-CPAP has been used to deliver a variable level of positive pressure to improve patient comfort. In theory, a variable level of pressure delivery could improve patient tolerance by limiting the delivered pressure.

Convincing data that auto-titrating devices improve patient outcome are currently lacking. Theoretically, however, this may be the ideal treatment for patients requiring variable pressures such as in REM-related apnoea.

Finally, communications with the bed partner about the importance of treatment for both neurocognitive and cardiovascular sequelae may also improve patient adherence.

The major problem with CPAP is compliance which is discussed above. Pressure sores around the nose and nasal crusting are usually minor and transient, and they are easily amenable to local therapies. Although discussed frequently, gastric insufflations and pneumothorax are rarely seen clinically.

Oral appliances

Several intraoral devices have been designed to enlarge the pharyngeal airway during sleep by moving either the tongue or the mandible anteriorally (Figure 10). Such devices are prepared by a dentist, and have been shown to enlarge the pharyngeal airway as measured by CT and MRI. Oral appliances appear to be very successful in improving snoring, but only partly successful at relieving apnoeas. In addition, the likelihood of success with an oral appliance appears to be inversely related to the

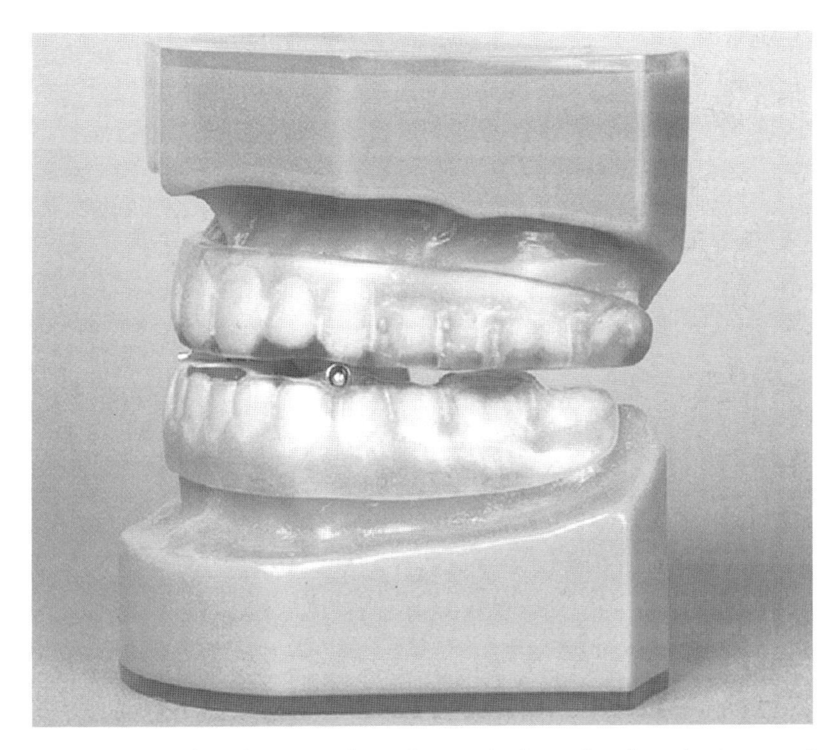

Figure 10 *Oral appliance used to advance the lower jaw in order to prevent apnoeas during sleep. Photograph courtesy of Alan A Lowe, Faculty of Dentistry, University of British Columbia.*

severity of apnoea, making them most useful for patients with a mild disease. In two randomized crossover trials of CPAP versus oral appliance therapy, CPAP was found to be more effective, especially in severe cases. However, patients preferred the oral appliance, despite some potential side effects.

Side effects of oral appliances are common but usually improve after the first 1–2 months. These include jaw discomfort, excessive salivation and sore teeth. However, a significant proportion of patients (60–65%) continue to complain of side effects after a 4-month treatment period, with approximately 20–24% classifying them as moderate to severe. Although no cases of permanent temperomandibular joint (TMJ) dysfunction have been reported, this is a theoretical concern. Therefore, oral appliances should be avoided in those with pre-existing TMJ dysfunction.

Upper airway surgery

It is estimated that no more than 2% of adults with OSA have a discrete anatomical abnormality of the upper airway which, if repaired, will lead to cure of the sleep apnoea. Thus, surgical approaches to treatment of sleep apnoea have been developed to enlarge the pharyngeal airway or bypass the obstruction. Tracheostomy was the first surgical procedure used in the treatment of apnoea, but currently it is rarely performed for sleep apnoea. Other procedures include radiofrequency (RF) ablation of the tongue or soft palate (somnoplasty), laser-assisted uvuloplasty (LAUP), uvulopalatopharyngoplasty (UPPP), or much more elaborate operations such as genioglossal advancement with hyoid myotomy, bimaxillary advancement or maxilomandibular advancement (MMA).

All of these aim to enlarge the pharyngeal airspace and consequently prevent airway collapse. Their success rate ranges from 30% for the less aggressive interventions to 90% in the most aggressive ones. Common side effects of UPPP include pain, alterations in taste and nasal regurgitation. The advantage of all surgeries is the potential for immediate benefit. The disadvantages, on the other hand, are the irreversible nature of the procedures, low success rate and relatively high occurrence of side effects.

Nasal treatment

Nasal pathology is associated with OSA. This may be related to increased negative pressure in the pharynx during inspiration as a result of the increased nasal resistance or interference with reflexes designed to protect the patency of the upper airway. Repair of nasal pathology has resulted in improvements of sleep apnoea, at least in the short term, in small case series. Thus, we should examine OSA patients for symptoms and signs of nasal pathology, and consider surgical or medical treatment if abnormalities are found. Surgical approach may include correction of deviated septum, polypectomy or turbinectomy. Medical approaches consist of daily use of decongestants (anticholinergics, steroids), which result in improvement in selected cases.

Pharmacological therapy

A variety of drugs has been used to treat OSA. These include respiratory stimulants, agents for increasing tone of the upper airway muscles and agents for treating hypersomnolence. Overall, pharmacological agents have been disappointing as a treatment option for OSA. Although use of supplemental oxygen in OSA results in substantial improvements in nocturnal desaturation and cardiac bradyarrhythmias, only modest reductions in the RDI are seen. In addition, hypersomnolence does not improve with oxygen therapy. Hence, oxygen cannot be considered as a first-line treatment for OSA, although it may be considered if significant hypoxaemia is present.

Medroxyprogesterone is a respiratory stimulant and has been used to treat OSA by increasing central neural drive to the pharyngeal muscles. At this time, progesterone cannot be considered an effective treatment for OSA, although it may play an adjunctive role in patients with the obesity hypoventilation syndrome. Protriptyline, a tricyclic antidepressant, has also been proposed as a treatment of OSA. Overall, it appears that it may modestly decrease the apnoea–hypopnoea index and oxygen desaturation. Although protriptyline may increase genioglossus tone (perhaps through its anticholinergic effect), the predominant mechanism is probably through its suppression of REM sleep, which is the stage of sleep during which OSA is usually the most severe. These drugs have a variety of side effects, including urinary retention, dry mouth and impotence. Therefore, although this drug may be a reasonable option in patients with predominately REM-associated OSA, the drug is often poorly tolerated as a result of the myriad adverse side effects.

Selective serotonin reuptake inhibitors (SSRIs) have been used in an attempt to diminish the reduction in upper airway muscle activity that occurs at sleep onset in OSA patients. Although animal studies have shown increased genioglossus muscle activity when serotonin activity is augmented on brain-stem preparations, there are limited data that this therapy is likely to benefit human patients with OSA. Although some small studies have shown modest reductions in RDI with SSRI treatment, most of the data indicate no major benefit. Thus, SSRIs cannot presently be recommended as a treatment option for OSA. Potential toxicities of SSRIs include insomnia, REM suppression, worsened periodic limb movements, increased appetite, the serotonin syndrome and hypomania.

Modafinil is a stimulant medication that is used to treat daytime sleepiness associated with narcolepsy. In OSA, use of modafinil resulted in improved daytime sleepiness and alertness; however, there is no effect on the frequency of sleep apnoeas. Therefore, as modafinil does not address the underlying pathophysiology of the disease, we cannot recommend this as primary or adjunctive treatment in OSA. Other drugs such as nicotine, theophylline, acetazolamide, naloxone, almitrine and bromocriptine are also ineffective in treating OSA. Salicylates have been shown to result in improved respiration in high doses, but side effects in these doses prevent it from being a treatment to consider.

OSA in children

In children, OSA is estimated to occur in 1–3%, although even higher prevalence has been reported, depending on the diagnostic criteria used. Obstructive sleep apnoea in children has many similarities to the adult syndrome, although as already noted there are some important differences. Male sex, which is an important risk factor in adults, seems not to play a role in children's OSA. Although in adults the ratio of men to women among OSA patients is as high as 5–10 : 1, it is approximately 1 : 1 in children. Another risk factor recognized in adults that is of lesser importance in children is increasing age. In children, the peak occurrence of OSA is between the ages of 2 and 5 years, which is the age when the tonsils and adenoids are at their largest in relation to the oropharyngeal size. It is clear that the most important risk factor for OSA in children is hypertrophy of the tonsils or adenoids. However, many other anatomical factors predisposing to OSA in children have been recognized, including choanal stenosis, nasal polyps, chronic nasal congestion, macroglossia, micrognathia, cleft palate repair, midface hypoplasia (e.g. Down's, Crouzon's and Apert's syndromes, achondroplasia), mandibular hypoplasia (e.g. Pierre–Robin sequence, Cornelia De Lange syndrome) or craniofacial trauma.

Symptoms in children are similar to those seen in adults, with the exceptions of restlessness, which is a more common symptom in children, and sleepiness, which is somewhat less of a problem compared with in adults. In children with OSA it is common that, paradoxically, despite sleepiness they demonstrate symptoms of attention deficit hyperactive disorder (ADHD). Severity criteria are different in children. Values are considered normal when the RDI is less than one event per hour, and the oxygen saturation does not fall to less than 92%. As the RDIs in children can be low despite a potentially severe disorder, recording of the end-tidal CO_2 is required. Hypercapnia (hypoventilation) of above 50 mmHg (6.7 kPa) is considered as sleep apnoea even in the absence of frank apnoeas or hypopnoeas. In addition, alternative severity criteria have been suggested. According to these criteria, grade 0 indicates normal children, grades 1–2 indicate simple snoring and increased upper airway resistance, respectively, grade 3 reflects apnoeas/hypopnoeas without oxygen desaturations and grade 4 with oxygen desaturations, and grade 5 with complications (e.g. cor pulmonale, cardiomegaly, heart failure).

Growth and development of children are dependent on sufficient sleep. Poor growth velocity associated with adequate caloric intake (failure to thrive) is a frequent consequence of OSA in children. The underlying mechanism is not well established but current hypotheses include the presence of a hypermetabolic state during sleep. It was recently reported that children with OSA demonstrate significant decrease in energy expenditure during sleep after an adenotonsillectomy. There was an increase in postoperative weight gain with no significant change in caloric intake. Other, less well-understood mechanisms contributing to it may be hypothalamic–pituitary hormonal changes (particularly decreased growth hormone secretion), diminished appetite (caused by alterations of taste and smell), difficulties in swallowing (resulting from kissing tonsils) or gastro-oesophageal reflux.

In a recent study low school performance was clearly associated with sleep disordered breathing (SDB), and treatment resulted in significant improvement in the children's achievements. Thus, poor growth as well as neurobehavioural and developmental consequences of OSA in children are well established, and should be avoided by early diagnosis and treatment of the disorder. Other potential consequences in children include secondary enuresis, which may resolve with appropriate treatment of OSA. Medical consequences, such as pulmonary and systemic hypertension, cor pulmonale or congestive heart failure, are also described in severe cases, but have been studied much more in adults than in children.

As childhood OSA is usually associated with adenotonsillar hypertrophy, most cases are amenable to surgical treatment. Adenotonsillectomy is the most common therapy for OSA in children, unless there is an identified underlying disease such as choanal stenosis, Pierre–Robin sequence, Crouzon's syndrome, etc. However, there is a subgroup of children with OSA without hypertrophy of tonsils or adenoids that cannot be ignored. Furthermore, studies have failed to show a correlation between OSA and the degree of adenotonsillar hypertrophy based on radiographic measurements, and in some children OSA persists after adenotonsillectomy. Finally, even children in whom OSA resolved after adenotonsillectomy may demonstrate recurrence during adolescence. Therefore, there is increasing paediatric experience with CPAP therapy when tonsillectomy and adenoidectomy are either unsuccessful or inappropriate.

Central sleep apnoea

Central sleep apnoea (CSA) is characterized by repeated episodes of apnoea during sleep, resulting from temporary loss of ventilatory effort. A central apnoea is conventionally defined as a period of at least 10 s without airflow, during which no ventilatory effort is evident. In this condition, unlike obstructive apnoea, both flow and respiratory effort are absent (Figure 11).

Diagnosis

The diagnosis of CSA generally requires a full night recording of standard PSG with a particular focus on respiratory effort. To prove that an apnoea is indeed central, it must be documented that there is no respiratory effort throughout the event. This is most effectively and consistently accomplished with either direct measurement of diaphragm contractions (diaphragmatic EMG) or an oesophageal balloon, and

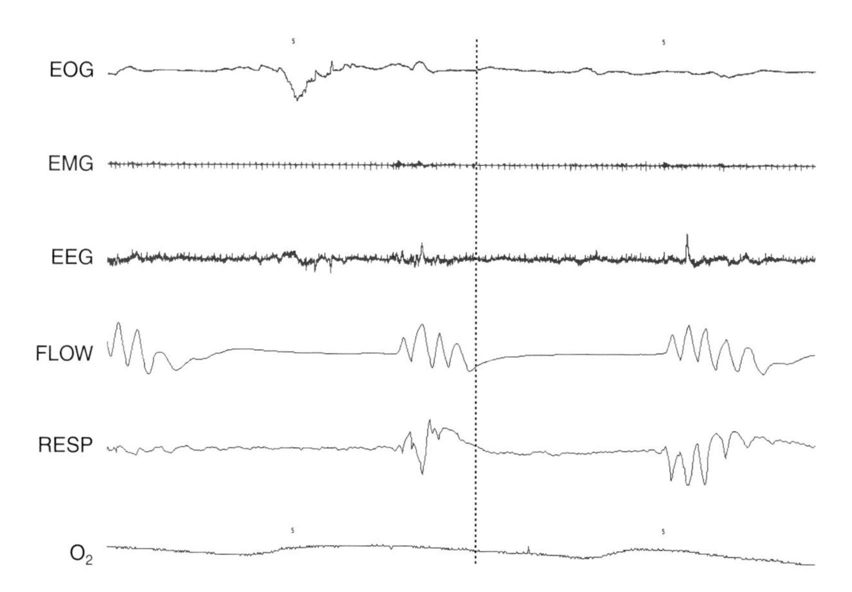

Figure 11 *An example of central sleep apnoeas (2 min). EOG, electrooculogram; EMG, electromyogram; EEG, electroencephalogram; Flow, airflow; RESP, respiratory effort; and O_2, oxygen saturation.*

direct measurements of intrathoracic pressures. However, both these techniques are cumbersome and invasive and may interfere with natural sleep more than the standard measurements. As a result, most clinical sleep laboratories do not use them; instead they measure respiratory efforts by abdominal belt or respiratory inductive plethysmography (RIP). Central apnoea is considered when there is a complete absence of thoraco-abdominal motion throughout an apnoea. Standard PSG is quite accurate in defining complete apnoea. However, distinguishing central from obstructive hypopnoeas is extraordinarily difficult and cannot reliably be accomplished using standard monitoring techniques. As a result, central apnoeas, rather than hypopnoeas, must be documented to make a definitive diagnosis of CSA. Moreover, as obstructive apnoeas are substantially more common than central events, most sleep laboratories require that at least 80% of the events will be of central origin in order to diagnose a patient with pure CSA.

As stated previously, five central apnoeas per hour of sleep are currently considered the upper limit of normal, and a greater frequency implies an abnormal state. As with obstructive apnoea, the severity of central apnoea is classified rather arbitrarily. As a result of the poor correlation between AHI and outcome, some question the use of this index in defining severity. Usually 5–20 events per hour of sleep with oxygen desaturations not lower than 85% is considered mild, 20–35 and O_2 desaturations no lower than 65% moderate, and more than that severe. Alternatively, severity may be determined by symptoms or complications. According to this, mild CSA is associated with mild insomnia or sleepiness and no complications, whereas for severe CSA severe sleepiness/insomnia is required and usually also cardiovascular complications.

Epidemiology

As there are no epidemiological studies aimed at finding the prevalence of CSA in the general population, only rough estimates are available. There are some reports of specific subtypes of CSA in specific populations, e.g. about 40% of patients with congestive heart failure (CHF) exhibit Cheyne–Stokes respiration (CSR) during sleep. CSR is a variant of central apnoea characterized by a waxing and waning pattern of breathing (see below). The overall prevalence of CSA in the general population is uncertain; from sleep laboratory populations, about 4–8% of patients with sleep apnoea syndrome have CSA. It is clearly more common in patients with neurological or cardiological abnormalities, as discussed below.

Pathophysiology

Before discussing the 'pure' CSA, it is important to mention that the distinction between CSA and OSA is not 'all or none', and frequently obstructive events are seen in CSA and vice versa, suggesting an overlap in the mechanisms responsible for the different types of apnoea. Furthermore, treatment of OSA by either tracheostomy or CPAP (particularly if the pressure is too high) may lead to the appearance of central apnoeas. Likewise, treating central apnoeas with either a respiratory stimulant (e.g. acetazolamide) or diaphragmatic pacing can result in obstructive events.

There are studies reporting narrowing of the pharyngeal airway during purely central apnoeas, so there are common features in the pathophysiology of the various types of apnoea. It is not therefore surprising that central and obstructive apnoeas are frequently seen in the same individual, a point of therapeutic relevance. In certain circumstances, a tendency towards upper airway obstruction may result in central ventilatory cycling.

Generally, CSA may be categorized into two groups: those with high waking P_{CO_2}, and those with normal or low waking P_{CO_2}, which differ in respect of their pathophysiology. Patients with waking hypercapnia may have diminished ventilatory response to hypercapnia and almost always demonstrate sleep-related hypoventilation and CSA. On the other hand, in patients with CSA without waking hypercapnia, the cause of the CSA may instead be increased ventilatory response to hypercapnia. During the wake–sleep transition, CO_2 level increases (e.g. from 40 mmHg to approximately 45 mmHg). In individuals with high ventilatory drive, a brief arousal (for whatever reason) may lead to a robust ventilatory response, driving down CO_2 to below the apnoea threshold 'overshoot'. The result is ventilatory control instability yielding periodic breathing (cycling) or CSA. Such cycling may occur with a variety of conditions associated with frequent awakenings from sleep. Thus, arousals from sleep are associated with temporary hyperventilation (post-arousal) and may lead to transient hypocapnia and subsequently apnoea.

Normal individuals who travel to high altitudes also display cyclic ventilation and CSA until habituation occurs. It should be noted, however, that CO_2 is not the only potential mechanism for ventilatory cycling; some researchers have suggested that increased tidal volume (vagal mechanisms), rather than low $P\text{CO}_2$, may be the primary mechanism inhibiting respiration after a series of large breaths (so-called neuromechanical inhibition). Regardless of the cause (secondary to hypocapnia or vagal mechanisms), the concept is that temporary hyperventilation ultimately leads to an inhibition of respiration with central apnoea. There are several additional potential components of periodic breathing and CSA, such as prolonged circulatory time (in CHF) or chemoreceptor abnormalities, as is discussed further under Cheyne–Stokes respiration. Table 19 outlines briefly some characteristics of the various types of CSA.

Nocturnal hypoventilation with waking hypercapnia (central alveolar hyperventilation syndrome, neuromuscular diseases, chronic lung diseases)

Generally, hypoventilation can result from neural origins (decreased ventilatory output), muscular reasons (respiratory muscle weakness) or pulmonary reasons (chronic restrictive or obstructive lung disease). Regardless of the cause, the system cannot maintain normal ventilation (i.e. eucapnia) during wakefulness, and this is typically worsened during sleep. As a result, the $P\text{CO}_2$ of these patients during sleep may reach extremely high levels, and this cycles around these levels (as opposed to much lower levels in the other types of CSA). Table 20 summarizes some of the more common diagnoses associated with CSA with waking hypercapnia. It should be emphasized, again, that many of them can be associated with obstructive apnoeas as well.

Table 19 Various types of central sleep apnoea

Condition	*Special features*
Idiopathic central sleep apnoea	Awake P_{CO_2} is normal or low Ventilatory hypercapnic response is normal or increased Commonly complain of insomnia and choking More common in men
Central alveolar hypoventilation syndrome	Awake hypoxaemia and hypercapnia that are worsened by sleep Worst during REM sleep Decreased ventilatory response to hypercapnia
Cheyne–Stokes respiration	Awake P_{CO_2} is normal or low Ventilatory hypercapnic response is normal or increased Common in neurological disorders and congestive heart failure
High-altitude associated respiratory cycling	Occurs in people acutely exposed to high altitude Awake P_{CO_2} is normal or low Ventilatory hypercapnic response is normal or increased Reduced during REM sleep

Central alveolar hypoventilation syndrome

The central alveolar hypoventilation syndrome (CAHS) is characterized by control of breathing abnormalities (low hypercapnic and hypoxic ventilatory responses) that lead to hypoventilation, which exist during wakefulness and are worsened during sleep. It was initially described in obese patients and was termed the 'obesity hypoventilation syndrome' (OHS), which is probably identical to the pickwickian syndrome. One of the first descriptions of the pickwickian syndrome was provided by Burwell and his colleagues in 1956. It consists of:

- Massive obesity
- Hypercapnia

Table 20 Diseases associated with central sleep apnoea and waking hypercapnia

Neurological
Stroke
Familial dysautonomia
Shy–Drager syndrome
Poliomyelitis
Parkinson's disease
Diabetes mellitus
Neuromuscular
Myasthenia gravis
Muscular
Myopathies (nemaline, metabolic)
Muscular dystrophies (Duchenne, myotonic dystrophy)
Myotonia congenita (Thomsen's disease)

- Hypersomnolence
- Hypoxaemia
- Polycythaemia
- Pulmonary hypertension
- Cor pulmonale.

However, in later years a similar syndrome was also described in non-obese patients, and in patients with OHS who still had impaired hypercapnic and hypoxic ventilatory responses after weight loss. Therefore, the current term is the 'central alveolar hypoventilation syndrome'. In the general population, this syndrome is quite rare, although it may affect as many as 10–15% of the morbidly obese patients (BMI > 40 kg/m^2). However, it should be mentioned that there is poor correlation between the degree of obesity and the occurrence of hypoventilation. This syndrome may also be secondary to CNS insults such as infarction, infection or demyelination. The CAHS syndrome should be distinguished from other causes of hypoventilation such as severe lung dysfunction or respiratory muscle weakness. Thus, a diagnosis of CAHS requires that pulmonary function and respiratory muscle force are not impaired.

Clinically, patients with CAHS may experience daytime hypercapnia and hypoxaemia that worsens during sleep, and deteriorates further during REM sleep. As a result, they may complain of sleep fragmentation and insomnia or hypersomnia, as well as morning headaches. In untreated patients the disorder may progress and be complicated by arrhythmias, pulmonary hypertension, cor pulmonale and heart failure. Treatment options include first and foremost weight loss. This may not change the ventilatory response to hypercapnia or hypoxaemia, but clearly improves the daytime profile of blood gases, as well as breathing during sleep and sleep consolidation. Other options include progesterone (respiratory stimulant), CPAP or BIPAP. Tracheostomy may be considered if other treatments fail.

High-altitude-associated respiratory cycling

It is well documented that humans acutely exposed to high altitude have periodic breathing during sleep with central apnoeas. This is a normal physiological response to the decreased oxygen tension rather than a specific pathology. It may result partially from the hypoxia that leads to hyperventilation; this results in hypocapnia and apnoea (if below the hypercapnic threshold). Indeed, it is most frequent in individuals who have a higher ventilatory response to hypoxia and hypercapnia. On subsequent nights, the periodic breathing diminishes, although in some individuals it may persist for several weeks. In some individuals acutely exposed to high altitude, periodic breathing may be noted even when awake, and further exacerbated during sleep. Interestingly, in contrast to all other types of apnoea that worsen during REM sleep, in these patients the regularity of respiration improves and stabilizes during REM sleep. This may partially result from the lower hypoxic ventilatory response during REM sleep.

Administration of either oxygen or CO_2 abolishes periodic breathing at high altitude, and has been shown to reduce arousals from sleep as well. However, whenever treatment of high altitude-induced CSA is indicated, usually a simpler choice is acetazolamide (see below for more details). Usually with time, humans habituate to the low oxygen tension at high altitude and local residents usually have normal breathing patterns without periodic breathing or CSA.

Cheyne–Stokes respiration

Cheyne–Stokes respiration is a unique breathing pattern usually characterized by three phases: a crescendo phase in which tidal volume increases gradually (with each breath) from hypopnoea to hyperpnoea, a decrescendo phase from hyperpnoea to hypopnoea and a frank central apnoea (see Figure 12). Thus, it is somewhat different from the idiopathic central apnoea that has a more abrupt onset and offset.

Cheyne–Stokes respiration is most commonly seen in patients with heart failure, but it has been reported in patients with neurological disorders and can also be seen without any notable underlying cause, particularly in elderly people (idiopathic). Pathophysiologically, patients with CSR tend to hyperventilate, and subsequently their $Pa\text{CO}_2$ falls below the apnoeic threshold, which triggers central apnoea. The tendency to hyperventilate in CHF patients is thought to result from the effects of pulmonary vagal afferent stimulation as a result of pulmonary venous congestion, although other factors may also be important (e.g. prolonged circulatory time caused by low cardiac output, increased ventilatory responsiveness to rising $P\text{CO}_2$). Furthermore, there is a correlation between the degree of CHF (ejection fraction) and the severity of CSR.

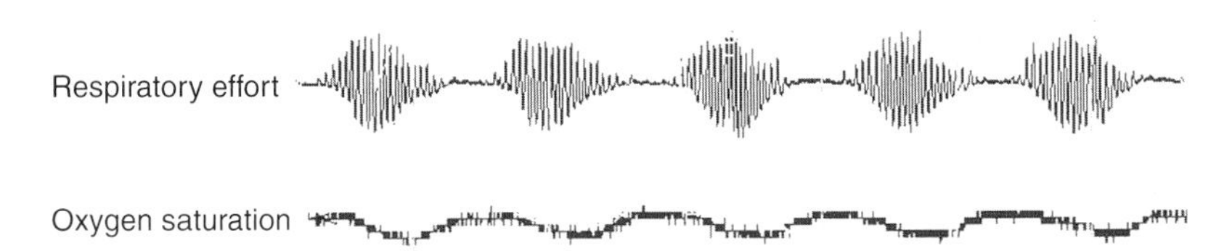

Figure 12 An example of Cheyne–Stokes respiration. Note the crescendo–decrescendo pattern of respiration, and the lag between hyperpnoea and increased oxygen saturation. This may result from the prolonged circulation time in patients with congestive heart failure, as the patient shown in this example (5 min).

The mechanism of CSR in patients with neurological abnormalities is less well understood. Regardless of the cause, patients with CSR demonstrate sleep fragmentation, with the arousals seen usually at the peak of the hyperpnoeic phase. This may result in daytime somnolence similar to OSA (see later). In addition, in patients with CHF, CSR may have great clinical importance with prognostic implications. Several studies have reported reduced survival in patients with left ventricular failure and CSR, compared with patients who have heart failure without CSR. Careful analyses have suggested that the apnoea–hypopnoea index is an independent predictor of mortality in CHF. Furthermore, it has been reported that treatment of CSR in CHF patients is associated with improved survival. However, it should again be mentioned that patients with CHF can frequently have a combination of both CSR (CSA) and OSA.

During the first night of CPAP treatment, the obstructive events are eliminated, although the central events may not be abolished. In this condition, a pressure of 10–12 cmH_2O has been shown to improve cardiovascular effects (increase left ventricular ejection fraction and reduce symptoms of heart failure) and also reduce the frequency of central apnoeas over time. Other signs of improvement with CPAP include fewer admissions to hospital, decrease in the degree of functional mitral regurgitation, lowered plasma atrial natriuretic peptide concentrations and reduced catecholamine concentrations (diurnal and nocturnal). Thus, other than optimizing medical treatment for the CHF, it appears that CPAP is the most beneficial therapy.

Clinical manifestations

The clinical presentation of patients with CSA depends on its cause. Patients with CAHS (waking hypercapnia) generally present with symptoms suggestive of respiratory failure. These include cor pulmonale, peripheral oedema and polycythaemia. However, restless sleep and daytime sleepiness are also commonly reported. Patients with CSA without waking hypercapnia, on the other hand, commonly present with choking or shortness of breath during sleep, restless sleep, and insomnia or daytime sleepiness. Patients with pure central apnoea (non-hypercapnic) are frequently not obese, and have less daytime hypersomnolence than patients with OSA. As the proportion of obstructive or mixed events increases in these patients (still with predominantly central apnoea), hypersomnolence may become more frequent.

Although these clinical symptoms do not correlate well with the degree of apnoea severity measured by the RDI, currently this is considered to be the marker of the disorder and its severity. Five central events per hour of sleep are considered the upper limit of normal. Thus, in order to diagnose sleep apnoea (both central and obstructive), polysomnography (PSG) is required. Another marker of apnoea from PSG is nocturnal arterial oxygen saturation. Desaturations occurring with central apnoeas are usually less severe than with obstructive events, possibly as a result of the ventilatory effort that occurs with obstructive apnoea but not with the central one, longer apnoea duration when obstructive, and reduced lung volume in patients with obstructive apnoea caused by obesity. Sleep in general is disrupted in patients with CSA, similarly to those with OSA, by both arousals caused by the respiratory disturbance and abnormal sleep architecture, with generally less deep sleep (stages 3–4) and REM sleep.

The acute hemodynamic consequences of central apnoeas have been poorly investigated. Nevertheless, it seems highly probable that, as with OSA, central apnoea with hypoxaemia and hypercapnia cause elevation in pulmonary pressure, with the hypercapnic, central apnoeic patients demonstrating more severe pressure elevations. Furthermore, the arousals from sleep and sympathetic surges may result in systemic hypertension similar to OSA. One factor distinguishing these two types of apnoea is that of negative intrathoracic pressure. During obstructive apnoea, highly negative intrathoracic pressures may be observed, yielding huge transmural left ventricular pressures. Thus ventricular wall stress or wall tension may be substantially greater in the presence of respiratory effort (OSA) compared with absent respiratory effort (CSA).

Treatment

As CSA is not a single disorder and may result from a variety of conditions, treatment should be individualized, based on the main features of the syndrome in a given patient. Usually, in patients with waking hypercapnia, the most appropriate treatment is nocturnal ventilation (pressure-cycle ventilation or BIPAP applied via nasal mask). For the non-hypercapnic CSA, a number of therapeutic options are available.

First, as stated earlier (see Pathophysiology), in CSA there may frequently also be obstructive events. In fact, in some cases actual obstructive events trigger CSA. In this proposed sequence, with the transition from wakefulness to sleep, the upper airway may obstruct (or partially obstruct), resulting in an obstructive apnoea (hypopnoea) and consequent arousal. It is well documented that arousals from sleep (not necessarily caused by respiratory abnormalities) result in hyperventilation for several seconds. Thus, obstructive apnoea can induce arousal which, in turn, results in hyperventilation and hypocapnia below the apnoeic threshold, and so respiratory cycling and central apnoeas occur. Therefore, any treatment for OSA (see later) may be beneficial for CSA as well. Specifically, if airway obstruction exists (anatomical, such as deflected nasal septum or enlarged tonsils, or functional, such as nasal congestion) it should be treated before considering the specific treatment for the CSA. Likewise, if other underlying causes for the CSA are identified (e.g. CHF), it should first be treated and thereafter the central apnoea reassessed.

Second, it should be kept in mind that these central apnoeas may be asymptomatic and may even resolve spontaneously in some patients. Thus, if the symptoms are not debilitating or other therapies fail, it is not inappropriate to follow some central apnoea patients.

Third, in pure CSA with no obvious underlying cause or when the treatment of the potential cause has failed, several therapeutic approaches exist. These are summarized in Table 21.

Acetazolamide (Diamox – a carbonic anhydrase inhibitor) is a respiratory stimulant known to produce a metabolic acidosis and probably a shift in the $P\text{CO}_2$ apnoeic threshold to a lower value. It has been shown to be effective in reducing central apnoea frequency in short-term usage (weeks), and potentially also in long-term usage. Interestingly, discontinuation of acetazolamide did not lead to an immediate return of symptoms or events. However, as stated previously, treatment of the central

Table 21 Potential treatments of central sleep apnoea

Treatment	*Daily dosage (mg)*	*Comments*
Acetazolamide	1000	Carbonic anhydrase inhibitor, resulting in diuresis and metabolic acidosis Contraindicated in marked renal or hepatic disease, and in glaucoma
Theophylline	5–10 mg/kg body weight	Adenosin receptor antagonist, phosphodiesterase inhibitor Effective in CSR Toxicity can cause arrhythmias, vertigo, convulsions, anorexia, agitation, irritability, headache
Naloxone	1–3	Opiate antagonist Respiratory stimulant May cause abstinence syndrome in addicted patients
Medroxy-progesterone	50–120	Increases ventilatory response to hypercapnia and hypoxia Can cause impotence, breast discomfort (worsen malignancy), hirsutism, alopecia, thromboembolism.
Clomipramine	10–100	Tricyclic antidepressant May reduce REM sleep and potentially activate upper airway muscle Side effects include constipation, dryness, urinary retention, blurred vision
Nasal CPAP	Pressure titrated	May reduce obstructive event and break cycling May increase CO_2 and reduce CSA Proved to be beneficial in CHF patients with CSR
Oxygen supplement	Titrated (low flow, 1–3 l/min)	May remove the initiating factor (as at altitude) and prevent the ventilatory depressant effect of hypoxia Improves oxygenation and may improve all types of CSA

CHF, congestive heart failure; CAPAP, computer-assisted positive airway pressure; CSA, central sleep apnoea; CSR, Cheyne–Stokes respiration.

events may result in obstructive ones. The explanation for this is unknown but may relate to the respiratory stimulating activity of acetazolamide in an individual with a collapsing airway during sleep. When little ventilatory effort is present, the apnoeas appear to be central. However, when respiration is stimulated, obstructive events develop. Clearly, follow-up sleep studies are necessary in patients being treated with acetazolamide.

Likewise, theophylline, another respiratory stimulant, may also improve CSA. This has been shown in patients with both CSA and CSR. In newborns and infants with CSA as a result of immaturity of the respiratory control system, this may be the drug of choice, but in adults it may be associated with significant adverse consequences and therefore will usually be reserved to use only if other options have failed.

Opiate drugs profoundly depress breathing, and the opioid antagonist naloxone is extremely effective in reversing the effects of morphines. For this reason, it has been tried in sleep apnoea patients. In OSA patients the results have been disappointing, but in central apnoeas it was mildly beneficial. Nevertheless, the data are sparse, and more reproducible controlled studies are needed. Currently, it is not considered a common practice to treat CSA with naloxone.

Medroxyprogesterone is a known respiratory stimulant. As a result, there are several studies examining the effects of this medication on sleep apnoea. Probably the best results have been reported in obese patients with the obesity hypoventilation syndrome. In these patients it resulted in improved sleep apnoea and improved waking arterial blood gas levels. Likewise, it has been shown to be effective in children with the Prader–Willi syndrome. However, in both OSA and idiopathic CSA the results were conflicting and disappointing. Furthermore, in men it can result in debilitating side effects. Thus, this is not considered as a realistic option for non-hypercapnic CSA.

Clomipramine is a tricyclic antidepressant that has had reported success in some CSA patients. The mechanism is unclear but may be related to the REM-suppressing effect of these medications, and may also be related to a potential upper airway muscle stimulation effect. However, once again it has not been studied extensively and it did not show reproducible beneficial results. This medication is also not considered a common treatment for sleep apnoea and may be reserved only for a few exceptional cases.

Nasal CPAP has been shown to be an effective therapy for some patients with CSA. Several potential mechanisms of action can be raised. First, as stated above, this will eliminate obstructive apnoea, which may be the precipitating factor for the central apnoeas. Second, CPAP may slightly increase the dead space and increase arterial CO_2 levels. This may be sufficient to keep CO_2 levels above the apnoeic threshold, and prevent the cycling and CSA. Third, CPAP increases in lung volume may increase oxygen stores and prevent hyperventilation mediated by hypoxaemia.

In addition, as mentioned, CPAP is considered to be the optimal treatment in patients with CHF and CSR, in whom optimization of medical therapy for the heart failure did not abolish the Cheyne–Stokes pattern of respiration. In these patients, CPAP improves cardiovascular effects (increases left ventricular ejection fraction and reduces symptoms of heart failure) and improves transplant-free survival. Thus, nasal CPAP should definitely be considered in patients with the various types of CSA. In the two mechanisms of action proposed, apnoeas should be abolished during the night of pressure titration spent in the laboratory. When CSR exists, CPAP may not abolish the apnoeas on the first night of titration. In these cases, a home therapeutic trial with a pressure of 10–12 cmH_2O should be initiated. It should be mentioned that there are several advanced 'smart' new CPAP devices, such as the computer-assisted positive airway pressure (CAPAP), which has recently been reported to abolish respiratory events in CHF patients with CSR on the first night of titration. This device increases pressure support during the hypopnoeic phase of CSR and provides timed back-up ventilation during the apnoeic phase of the CSR cycle. As a result of its immediate improvement in respiration, sleep quality and oxygenation, it is proposed that compliance with treatment will increase, although clinical trials are needed to prove this.

Supplemental oxygen has also been shown to improve CSA. Although the mechanism by which oxygen administration reduces central apnoeas has not yet been established, two explanations seem possible. One relates to the potential destabilizing influence of the hypoxic ventilatory response on respiratory control. This is best exemplified by the high altitude-related CSA. If the initial factor is removed (i.e. alveolar hypoxia), this may prevent the resulting hyperventilation and hypocapnia, which results in cycling and CSA. The other potential mechanism of action is based on the observation that hypoxia can be a ventilatory depressant. If respiration is depressed by hypoxia, then central apnoeas may occur. Oxygen administration in this situation could reduce apnoeas. Whatever the mechanism, low-flow oxygen may be an effective treatment for CSA. This has been shown specifically in CHF patients with Cheyne–Stokes breathing, in whom it reduced the frequency of apnoea and improved the symptoms.

However, unlike CPAP, oxygen supplementation has not been shown to improve survival in CSR patients and in fact some researchers believe that oxygen may have adverse effects on patients with CHF and CSR as a result of its potential to produce free radicals. Thus, oxygen treatment is absolutely considered a viable treatment for patients with all forms of CSA, although it seems that nasal CPAP may be superior and should be offered first. This is especially the case in the vast majority of central apnoea patients in whom both central and obstructive apnoeas are commonly seen in the same individual. Thus, treatment of the airway obstruction may have beneficial effects on both types of apnoea.

chapter 5

Periodic limb movement disorder

> You will see mettlesome steeds, when their limbs are at rest, still continuing in sleep to sweat and pant as if straining all their strength to win the palm, or as if the lifted barriers of the starting-post had just released them. And the huntsman's hounds, while wrapped in gentle slumber, often toss their legs with a quick jerk and utter sudden whines and draw rapid breaths of air into their nostrils as if they were hot on a newly-found scent.
>
> Lucretius, *De Rerum Natura (On the Nature of the Universe)*, 1 BC. Latham RE (trans.) Baltimore: Penguin, 1959.

Periodic limb movement disorder (PLMD), also known as nocturnal myoclonus or periodic movements in sleep, is a disorder of intermittent movements of the extremities during sleep. It usually affects the legs, but occasionally the arms. The movements are periodic, highly stereotypical, and may or may not be associated with arousals from sleep. As PLMD frequently causes sleep fragmentation and consequently nocturnal insomnia, we also discuss it in Chapter 8. When it exists without arousals or sleepiness, however, it may be classified under undesired movements during sleep (see Chapter 8).

Characteristics and clinical features

The most typical movements are extension of the hallux and/or partial or complete dorsiflexion of the foot at the ankle. Infrequently it may include movements of the knee, rarely the hip and sometimes the arm. The patients themselves usually do not remember the leg movements, although occasionally they may complain of muscular pain in the morning. The more likely clinical complaint of PLMD is daytime somnolence, resulting from the sleep fragmentation. Sometimes the suspicion is raised based on an observer's (spouse's) report, and the patient is asymptomatic. Less frequently the movements may result in awakenings and sleep maintenance insomnia.

Diagnosis

The diagnosis of PLMD is laboratory based rather than clinical. It requires a full night polysomnographic sleep study, which demonstrates the characteristic limb movements. Surface electrodes are usually placed over the anterior tibialis muscle (lateral calf), but sometimes upper limbs are also monitored (if clinically indicated). Anterior tibialis electromyography (EMG) of every movement demonstrates contractions lasting 0.5–5 s. A leg movement is considered part of a PLM sequence if it is a part of at least four movements separated by more than 5 s and less than 90 s. If more than 90 s separates two movements, they will not be grouped together, and if fewer than four movements are encountered in a given series, these movements will be considered sporadic and not periodic, and will not be counted as PLMs. The movements may affect one or both legs, usually in an unpredictable fashion (e.g. movements may occur in left, right or both feet in a seemingly random order). Simultaneous movements in both legs are counted as one. Examples of PLMs in a six minute segment from a polysomnography are shown in Figure 13. Leg movements resulting from arousals caused by respiratory disturbances are not counted as PLMs.

Based on these criteria, the total nocturnal periodic movements are

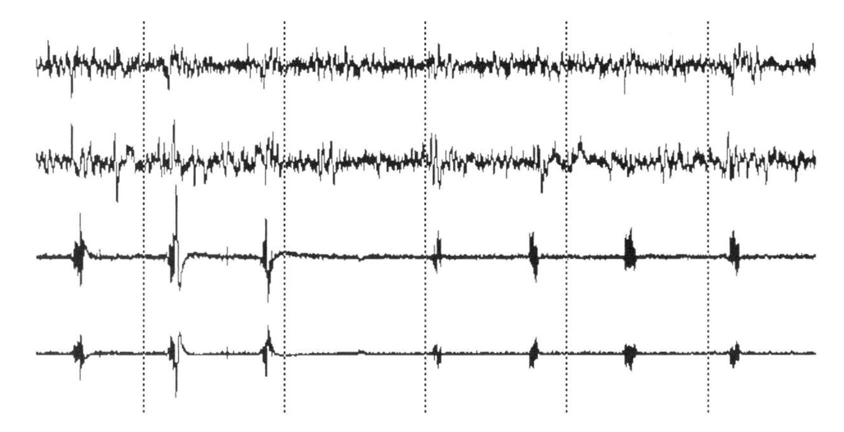

Figure 13 *An example of periodic leg movements (PLMs) in sleep (6 min). Two channels of EEG and electromyogram from the left and right legs.*

counted. The periodic limb movement index (PLMI) is computed by dividing the total number of PLMs by the total sleep time in hours (the number of periodic movements per hour of sleep). Based on the PLMI, and the portion of the movements that causes arousals, the severity is determined. Up to five periodic movements per hour of sleep are considered normal. A PLMI of 5–24/h indicates mild PLMD, 25–49/h is considered moderate and 50/h or more indicates severe PLMD. If there are 25 or more periodic movements per hour of sleep, which are associated with arousals from sleep, the disorder is considered to be severe. However, these cut-offs are rather arbitrary, necessitating clinical judgement in the management of individual patients.

An additional polysomnographic finding in PLMs is the relatively frequent occurrence of movements in NREM sleep (especially in stage 2 sleep, and less common in stages 3–4), and relatively rare in REM sleep. For this reason, and potentially for circadian modulation as well, PLMs seem to occur more frequently in the first rather than in the second half of the night.

One limitation of a single-night sleep study is the relatively high night-to-night variability in PLMs. Therefore, when PLMD is clinically strongly suspected and polysomnography does not reveal PLMs, a second diagnostic night may be indicated.

Aetiology and risk factors

The cause of PLMD is unknown. The pathophysiology may involve vascular and/or peripheral and central nervous system (CNS) abnormalities. The strongest data suggest involvement of the dopaminergic system, with some modulation of the opioid system. As a cortical locus for PLMD has not been found despite attempts, a subcortical location is probably responsible for generating these movements. Furthermore, as PLMD increases with spinal cord injuries, and can be induced in animals with complete transection of the spinal cord, the oscillator generating the stereotypical movements in PLMD may be located within the spinal cord.

There are several clinical conditions associated with periodic limb movements (PLMs). These include the use of medications such as tricyclic antidepressants or selective serotonin reuptake inhibitors (SSRIs), or withdrawal of medications such as anticonvulsants, barbiturates or other hypnotics. Excess of caffeinated beverages is also well known to increase PLMD. In addition, PLMD is common in some medical conditions such as renal failure and Parkinson's disease. Some proportion of patients with PLMD also have restless leg syndrome (RLS), but most of the patients with RLS (80%) have PLMD. Thus, risk factors for RLS (e.g. peripheral neuropathy, low iron stores) are also important in PLMD. As RLS is primarily a clinical disorder associated with difficulties initiating and maintaining sleep, it is discussed in Chapter 7.

Age also plays a role in PLMD. Generally, it is uncommon in childhood and increases with age (see below). Finally, some reports support familial aggregation of PLMs although there are insufficient data to support a specific mode of inheritance.

Epidemiology

The prevalence of PLMD is estimated to be about 5% in the general population, and increases dramatically with age, especially after 50 years of age. In children it is considered to be quite rare, although recent work reveals that it may be relatively common (10%) in children with attention deficit disorder. In elderly people, on the other hand, PLMD becomes very common. The prevalence of PLMD has been reported to be 20–44% in patients aged over 60 years, and 58% in those aged over 65 years. There appears to be no sex predisposition. The prevalence may be very high in high-risk groups such as patients with chronic renal failure and uraemia.

Differential diagnosis

> Wherefore to some, when being a Bed, they betake themselves to sleep, presently in the arms and legs, leaping and contractions of the tendons, and so great a restlessness and Tossing of their members ensue, that the diseased are no more able to sleep, than if they were in a Place of the greatest Torture.
>
> Thomas Willis, *Practice of Physick*. Pordage S (trans.) London, 1684.

The two main symptoms of PLMD are excessive daytime sleepiness and undesired limb movements during sleep. Thus, it should be distinguished from other causes of excessive daytime somnolence (EDS) and/or other causes of movements during sleep. The history is usually sufficient to distinguish PLMD from obstructive sleep apnoea or narcolepsy. Occasionally, EDS seems to be idiopathic, based on the history, and only during polysomnography is PLMD diagnosed. Similarly, when the presenting symptom is undesired movements during sleep, history alone may sometimes not be sufficient to make the diagnosis, and polysomnography is required. PLMD is usually easy to distinguish from some normal movement phenomena such as sleep starts (seen during wake–sleep transitions, with no periodic fashion) or phasic REM movements (occurs exclusively during REM sleep and is also non-periodic). Rhythmic movement disorder, seizure-related movements, REM sleep behaviour disorder and sleep walking all have different characteristics, and can easily be distinguished from PLMD, usually by history alone, but sometimes exclusively by polysomnography.

Treatment

The initial treatment for PLMD would be elimination of potential underlying causes, e.g. discontinuation of SSRIs, withdrawal from caffeine or correction of iron deficiency anaemia will often result in symptomatic improvement. As iron is important in dopamine biosynthesis and in dopamine receptors, some advocate doing complete iron tests (haemoglobin, ferritin, transferrin saturation) in all PLMD patients. Some patients without overt iron deficiency anaemia will respond to iron supplementation. Otherwise, generally, the treatment of PLMD is pharmacological, although some other treatments such as behavioural (moderate exercise, hot baths), herbal, nutritional (vitamins or minerals), and electrical foot stimulations, have been anecdotally proposed.

The effective medications improving PLMD can be categorized into four groups (Table 22): dopaminergic, benzodiazepine, opioid and others (including anticonvulsants, anti-adrenergics and muscle relaxants).

The goal of therapy for PLMD is usually to consolidate sleep, and consequently to improve daytime alertness. Occasionally, when movements and restless sleep are the chief complaint (by the partner), the goal may be to reduce the movements. It is generally considered that dopaminergic treatment has the potential to reduce the movements, although some sleep disruption may still exist. Treatment with benzodiazepines or opioids may be superior in consolidating sleep, although some movements may still occur. This distinction is not clear cut and the literature consists of conflicting data, sometimes showing reduction of movements with hypnotic therapy and improvement of sleep architecture with dopaminergic treatment. In fact, there are some papers reporting significant improvement of sleep architecture, PLM events and PLM-associated arousals, which were even significantly better with dopaminergic agonists compared with opioids.

It should be mentioned, however, that most papers reported short-term

Table 22 Pharmacological agents for the treatment of restless leg syndrome/periodic leg movements

Group	*Medication*	*Dosage range (mg)*
Dopaminergics	L-Dopa/carbidopa	25/100–50/200
	Pergolide	0.125–0.75
	Bromocriptine	2.5–10
	Pramipexole	0.125–0.50
Hypnotics	Clonazepam	0.5–2.0
	Lorazepam	0.5–2.0
	Triazolam	0.125–0.25
	Temazepam	15–60
Opioids	Morphine (sustained release)	15–30
	Methadone	10–30
	Oxycodone (sustained release)	10–40
	Propoxyphene	20–80
Others	Carbamazepine	100–400
	Gabapentin	300–2000
	Propranolol	40–160
	Clonidine	0.1–0.5
	Baclofen	20–80
	Iron	15–100

follow-up of patients on this treatment, and relatively little is known about the long-term consequences of treatment. A number of important complications of treatment have been reported, especially with the use of the dopaminergic agonists. These include mainly the rebound phenomenon (increase of PLMs in the second part of the night, when they were usually mild or absent) and the augmentation phenomenon (worsening of RLS/PLMD with long-term use of medications). These were noted primarily with the short-acting dopaminergic medications. Recent evidence suggests that long-acting dopaminergics (e.g. long-acting L-dopa/carbidopa [Sinemet CR] and pramipexole [Mirapex]) provide optimal relief of symptoms and improvement in sleep quality, with relatively mild or no side effects.

The well-known complications in patients treated with dopaminergic agonists for Parkinson's disease (e.g. dyskinesias) have not been reported when the indication was RLS/PLMD even with prolonged (years) treatment. Some side effects of dopaminergics, however, should be kept in mind (e.g. headaches with pergolide, hypotension with bromocriptine, nausea with pramipexole). The major side effects of the benzodiazepines are sleepiness, 'hang-over' the following day and, potentially, falls in elderly people. There are some recent data suggesting an increased risk of road traffic accidents among patients who use benzodiazepines chronically. Similar side effects can be seen with the opioids, with the addition of constipation. Table 22 summarizes the medications that have been used for RLS/PLMD. Generally, the first-line therapy should be a long half-life dopaminergic or a benzodiazepine. The other option would usually be tried only if the former did not work, or was associated with side effects, or if there is a contraindication to its use.

chapter 6

Primary and other forms of hypersomnia

Narcolepsy

Narcolepsy is a relatively rare disorder with a prevalence of 0.02–0.05%, depending on the population studied. It may be more frequent in Japan (prevalence of 0.18%) and is very rare in Israel (0.002%). It is manifested by abnormal sleepiness, disturbed nocturnal sleep and pathological manifestations of REM sleep. In the 1930s, Daniels described the classic tetrad of daytime sleepiness, cataplexy, sleep paralysis and hypnagogic hallucinations. The onset of clinical manifestations of narcolepsy, although variable, are typically during the second decade of life. The primary symptom is excessive sleepiness, which manifests itself as irresistible episodes of drowsiness or sleep that occur both during monotonous activities and when actively engaged. The sleepiness is classically relieved by brief naps, from which the patient awakens feeling refreshed, only to have sleepiness return within several hours. The other commonly associated symptoms represent manifestations of abnormal REM sleep.

Cataplexy, a 'breakthrough' of REM atonia into wakefulness, is the abrupt, reversible loss of muscle tone, usually triggered by a strong emotion such as laughter or anger. Typically this affects postural muscles, and severity can range from mild sagging of the jaw and weakness of the knees, to collapse from complete paralysis. These episodes may last from seconds to several minutes and consciousness is usually maintained. Although cataplexy has been traditionally considered as a 'breakthrough' of REM sleep atonia, recent studies in canine narcolepsy suggest that mechanisms and brain-stem sites for triggering cataplexy are not identical to those regulating REM sleep. Two additional classic symptoms result from REM-sleep related abnormalities. These include sleep paralysis (a transient inability to move or speak at awakening or falling asleep) and hypnagogic hallucinations (simple or complex hallucinatory experiences at sleep onset). In addition to these classic symptoms, other common features of narcolepsy include fragmented sleep and automatic behaviour during sleep such as sleep talking or walking (see Chapter 8). Sleep laboratory investigation is very helpful in diagnosing narcolepsy, although it is not an obligatory requirement. Classic clinical manifestations are sufficient to make the diagnosis without laboratory studies, as detailed in Table 23.

There is a clear familial tendency for narcolepsy. The risk of a first-degree relative of someone with narcolepsy developing narcolepsy is 1–2%, a 10–40 times higher risk than in the general population. Nevertheless, most of the cases are sporadic. Moreover, most monozygotic twin pairs have been found to be discordant for narcolepsy. Thus, environmental factors must also play a role in the development of narcolepsy, and may include head trauma, infections or other yet to be discovered factors.

This is the opposite of the clear autosomal recessive inheritance with full penetrance observed in narcoleptic Dobermans and Labradors. In these two species, narcolepsy has recently been found to be caused by a mutation in the hypocretin-2 receptor gene (*Hcrtr 2*). Hypocretins or orexins are novel neuropeptides localized within the lateral hypothalamus. The different nomenclature results from the simple fact that they were discovered at the same time by two different groups, and were named differently. They were initially believed mostly to control appetite (*orexin* means appetite in Greek), but they are now believed to have other functions such as regulatory effects on blood pressure, body temperature and the sleep–wake cycle. Indeed, neurons in the lateral hypothalamus are known to be involved in the maintenance of the waking state. The mutations found in the *Hcrtr 2* most probably cause impairment of post-

Table 23 Diagnostic criteria of narcolepsy based on ICSD (347)

A	A complaint of excessive sleepiness or sudden muscle weakness	
B	Recurrent daytime naps or lapses into sleep that occur almost daily for at least 3 months	
C	Sudden bilateral loss of postural muscle tone in association with intense emotion (cataplexy)	
D	Associated features include:	
	1	Sleep paralysis
	2	Hypnagogic hallucinations
	3	Automatic behaviours
	4	Disrupted major sleep episode
E	Polysomnography demonstrates one or more of the following:	
	1	Sleep latency <10 min
	2	REM latency <20 min
	3	An MSLT that demonstrates a mean sleep latency of <5 min
	4	Two or more sleep-onset REM periods
F	HLA (human leukocyte antigen) typing demonstrates DR2 positivity	
G	Absence of any medical or psychiatric disorder that could account for the symptoms	
H	Other sleep disorders may be present but are not the primary cause of the symptoms, e.g. periodic limb movement disorder or central sleep apnoea syndrome.	

Minimal criteria: B + C, A + D + E + G

synaptic hypocretin neurotransmission. At the same time it was found that pre-pro-hypocretin (pre-pro-orexin) knockout mice also exhibit a narcoleptic phenotype. Thus, deficits in either the hypocretin ligand or its receptor cause narcolepsy in animal models. Although inheritance in humans is not a simple mendelian one, hypocretin may play a role in human narcolepsy as well. It was recently reported that seven of nine narcoleptic patients had undetectable levels of hypocretin in their cerebrospinal fluid (CSF), as opposed to eight controls who had normal hypocretin levels.

In humans, narcolepsy has been linked to the class II MHC (major histocompatibility complex) antigen DR2, which was initially found in more than 90% of patients who had narcolepsy with cataplexy. Subsequent work has shown that DQB1*0602 is the most frequent haplotype associated with narcolepsy, being more sensitive than DR2. However, human leukocyte antigen (HLA) typing is of limited value in clinical practice. First, the HLA association is very high (>90%) only in narcoleptic patients with definite cataplexy, when diagnosis can be made by history only. Many patients with doubtful cataplexy are DQB1*0602 negative, dropping the sensitivity of this HLA marker to 40–60%. Second, the specificity of HLA typing is not high because DQB1*0602 is present in approximately 25% of the general population (range between 12 and 34%, depending on the population). In addition, from the mechanistic point of view, the role of HLA antigens in narcolepsy is unclear. HLA class II molecules (DR, DQ and DP) play a pivotal role in the genetic control of normal and pathological immune responses. It is therefore possible that an autoimmune process might be involved in the pathophysiology of narcolepsy, but this has not been found. Thus, it appears that, despite the close association with HLA alleles, narcolepsy in most humans is polygenic, with environmental factors also playing a role.

There is no specific treatment for narcolepsy, rather the treatment is symptomatic, and thus can be separated into the treatment of excessive sleepiness and the prevention of cataplexy. Non-pharmacological measures include adequate nocturnal sleep to prevent sleep deprivation, along with one to two short (30-min) daytime naps, if possible. Regular napping usually relieves sleepiness on a short-term basis, although frequently it cannot be achieved because of the negative social and professional consequences. A supportive social environment, such as patient organizations, is helpful as well. In most patients, however, non-pharmacological treatment is not sufficient and medications are required.

Pharmacological therapy of excessive daytime somnolence involves CNS-stimulant drugs (Table 24). The amphetamine-like agents (amphetamine, methylphenidate, pemoline) all work by increasing monoaminergic transmission in the CNS (mainly dopamine and norepinephrine/noradrenaline). Modafinil (provigil) is a novel agent

Table 24 Commonly used stimulant medications

Medication	*Dose (mg/day)*	*Side effects*
Methylphenidate	20–80	Tachycardia, hypertension, irritability, decreased appetite, insomnia, tolerance
Dextroamphetamine	15–60	Tachycardia, hypertension, irritability, decreased appetite, insomnia, tolerance
Pemoline	75–150	Tachycardia, hypertension, irritability, decreased appetite, insomnia, tolerance, liver toxicity
Modafinil	100–400	Headaches

that promotes wakefulness and is chemically distinct from the other stimulants. Its mode of action is not completely understood. Its major advantages appear to include a lower incidence of side effects and less potential for abuse, although it may not be as potent as some of the older stimulants. The most widely used medication currently is methylphenidate, probably because of the combination of high potency and short half-life (3–4 h), which allows patients to use it on an 'as needed' basis, while still having the option of napping. Pemoline and Modafinil have relatively long half-lives (approximately 16 and 12 h, respectively). The strategy of pharmacological treatment is usually to use the lowest effective dosage. Patients are instructed to begin with a low dose, and increase the dosage as needed to achieve clinical satisfaction. Tolerance may develop and drug holidays may be indicated. The final dosage is frequently a compromise between efficacy and side effects, such as headaches, irritability, anorexia, palpitations and some gastric discomfort, which often develop.

Cataplexy is treated with drugs that are known to suppress REM sleep, including the tricyclic antidepressants and selective serotonin reuptake inhibitors (SSRIs) (Table 25). Although the tricyclics are probably more potent REM suppressors, they are generally less well tolerated. Most of them have strong anticholinergic side effects, leading to dry mouth,

Table 25 Antidepressants commonly used to alleviate cataplexy and other REM-related symptoms

Medication	*Dose (mg/day)*	*Side effects*
Fluoxetine	20–40	Sleep disturbances, periodic limb movements, sexual dysfunction
Paroxetine	20–40	Sleep disturbances, periodic limb movements, sexual dysfunction
Sertraline	50–150	Sleep disturbances, periodic limb movements, sexual dysfunction
Clomipramine	25–75	Nausea, dry mouth, constipation, tremor, urinary retention, arrhythmias
Desipramine	50–150	Nausea, dry mouth, constipation, tremor, urinary retention, arrhythmias
Nortriptyline	50–100	Nausea, dry mouth, constipation, tremor, urinary retention, arrhythmias
Protriptyline	15–20	Nausea, dry mouth, constipation, tremor, urinary retention, arrhythmias
Imipramine	75–150	Nausea, dry mouth, constipation, tremor, urinary retention, arrhythmias

constipation, urinary retention, tachycardia, blurred vision and potentially orthostatic hypotension (resulting from α_1-adrenergic blockade) and severe cardiac arrhythmias (mainly with intoxication). Additional side effects of tricyclics may include weight gain, sexual dysfunction, tremors, and potentially sedation caused by antihistaminic effects. Sometimes they may promote sleep fragmentation, mainly as a result of enhancement of periodic limb movements in sleep, although worsening of periodic limb movements is more frequently seen with the use of SSRIs. Thus, commonly, the treatment of choice is an SSRI (frequently fluoxetine).

Additional symptoms sometimes needing treatment are sleep paralysis, sleep disruption and hypnagogic hallucinations. As sleep paralysis and hypnagogic hallucinations are manifestations of REM sleep, frequently the antidepressants that alleviate cataplexy may also be beneficial to these. However, the SSRIs can worsen nocturnal sleep, fragmentation of which is characteristic of narcolepsy. Thus, some of these patients may benefit paradoxically from short half-life hypnotic medications, which have been shown to consolidate nocturnal sleep and reduce excessive daytime somnolence and even cataplexy. One example of such a medication is γ-hydroxybutyrate.

Idiopathic hypersomnia

Idiopathic hypersomnia (IH), also called idiopathic CNS hypersomnia, is characterized by excessive sleepiness without any identifiable cause. Nocturnal sleep is usually long and undisturbed, and there is no other finding that can explain the sleepiness, such as head trauma, anaemia, hypothyroidism, etc. It is assumed that there is a CNS abnormality (of the sleep–wake mechanisms), yet unrecognized, that causes the sleepiness. This syndrome has had a number of labels, including essential narcolepsy, independent narcolepsy, functional hypersomnia and harmonious hypersomnia. The *International Classification of Sleep Disorders* defined IH as 'a disorder of presumed central nervous system cause that is associated with normal or prolonged major sleep episodes, and excessive sleepiness consisting of prolonged (1–2 hours) sleep episodes of non-REM sleep'. The age of onset of the syndrome is usually late adolescence, and there is no clear sex predisposition.

The exact prevalence of the syndrome is unknown, but is estimated to be 2–5 per 100 000 (0.002–0.005%). It accounts for 1–10% of patients who are referred to sleep clinics because of daytime sleepiness. Clinical observations support familial manifestation of IH, but genetic studies have failed to show specific gene association. Furthermore, HLA studies in IH were also inconclusive, although some reports have shown high frequency of HLA-DR5, -Cw2 and -B27 among these patients.

The syndrome of idiopathic CNS hypersomnia is less well defined and understood than narcolepsy. The major clinical characteristics include prolonged nocturnal sleep episodes, difficulty awakening from sleep (also referred to as 'sleep inertia' or 'sleep drunkenness') and often, long unrefreshing naps. The abrupt sleep attacks and symptoms of abnormal REM sleep seen in narcolepsy are absent. As there is no direct positive diagnosis, the diagnosis is made by exclusion of other causes of excessive daytime sleepiness, including sleep apnoea, periodic limb movements, narcolepsy, insufficient sleep, long sleeper and affective disorder. Thus, to make this diagnosis, polysomnography followed by an MSLT is essential. Polysomnography typically reveals normal sleep architecture and increased sleep efficiency. Sometimes increased slow wave sleep is observed. MSLT reveals a shortened sleep-onset latency (≤8 min), usually without sleep onset REMs (SOREMs). It may be difficult to distinguish idiopathic CNS hypersomnia from narcolepsy without cataplexy, because not all those with narcolepsy will reveal ≥2 SOREMs at initial MSLT. The presence of HLA-DQB1*0602 may therefore be helpful. Treatment consists of the use of stimulant medications (see Table 24), although, unlike narcolepsy (see Table 26), IH patients sometimes respond less favourably to stimulants and experience more side effects. Naps are often not refreshing in these patients; however, obtaining regular nocturnal sleep may help minimize symptoms.

Table 26 The common and differentiating factors of narcolepsy and idiopathic hypersomnia

	Narcolepsy	*Idiopathic hypersomnia*
EDS	Yes	Yes
Naps	Refreshing	Frequently not refreshing
Cataplexy	Yes	No
Awakenings	Refreshed (for a while)	Commonly 'sleep inertia'
HH, SP	Frequently	No
PSG	Fragmented sleep	Sleep is not disrupted
MSLT	<5 min, ≥2 SOREMs	<5 min, no SOREMs
HLA	DQB1*0602	CW2 (?)
Stimulants	Beneficial, well tolerated	Unpredictable response

EDS, excessive daytime somnolence; HH, hypnagogic hallucinations; SP, sleep paralysis; PSG, polysomnography; MSLT, multiple sleep latency test.

Recurrent hypersomnolence

Recurrent hypersomnia, also known as periodic hypersomnia, is a disorder of excessive sleepiness that occurs in periods, with each episode lasting several days to several weeks; it may occur up to 12 times a year, although usually the frequency is one or two episodes per year. During an episode, the patient is extremely sleepy and can sleep as much as 20 hours per day, waking up only for eating and voiding. It has been reported to occur after trauma or viral infections such as Epstein–Barr virus (EBV) or cytomegalovirus (CMV), but the more frequent finding is recurrent hypersomnia of unknown aetiology, better known as the Kleine–Levin syndrome (KLS). This is a rare but probably underdiagnosed disorder affecting mainly adolescent boys and young men. It is characterized by periodic episodes of hypersomnia, accompanied frequently by hyperphagia (compulsive eating) and abnormal behaviour that may include features of hypersexuality (e.g. patients may find themselves masturbating in the living room even if other people are around, or may touch strangers inappropriately). Patients can gain several kilograms in weight during an episode. They may experience depression, depersonalization, aggression, irritability and hallucinations during the attacks. However, neither hyperphagia nor abnormal behaviour or mental changes are required to make the diagnosis, although their existence makes the diagnosis relatively clear.

Episodes may be precipitated by febrile disease, strong emotions or stress. Table 27 presents some of the clinical features of 34 male KLS patients seen in the Technion sleep laboratory over the years. On sleep laboratory polysomnographic examination, during an episode, the patients demonstrate long sleep with high sleep efficiency, although there is increased sleep fragmentation and somewhat reduced stages 3 and 4 sleep. MSLT reveals short sleep latencies, potentially with one or more SOREMs. Between the episodes of sleepiness, the patients are completely normal, both physically and mentally. They are not sleepy and their behaviour is normal. Investigational studies between episodes such as polysomnography, MSLT, computed tomography of the brain, full-montage EEG, etc. reveal normal findings. The disorder apparently

Table 27 Characteristics of 34 male patients with Kleine–Levin syndrome

	Mean ± SD	*Range*
Onset (years)	15.8 ± 2.8	9–21
Diagnostic delay (years)	3.8 ± 4.2	0.5–14
Duration of attack (days)	11.5 ± 6.6	3–42
Number of attacks	7.5 ± 6.2	2–25
Precipitating factors	16/34 patients (47%)	Fever (12); hot climate (3); anxiety state (1)

decreases with age and remits spontaneously, yielding an excellent prognosis. The frequency, severity and duration of the episodes decrease until they cease completely at mid to late adulthood. There is no specific treatment. Therapy should be individualized and be primarily supportive (including safety and protective measures). Stimulants may potentially alleviate sleepiness, although there are insufficient data to support their use. Furthermore, it remains unclear whether any treatment alters the natural history of this disorder (i.e. shortens episodes or decreases their frequency).

Post-traumatic hypersomnolence

This syndrome consists of symptoms and signs of hypersomnia, which are generally very similar to IH, except that they develop following head trauma. Although there are several cases reporting full-blown, narcolepsy-like syndrome developing after head trauma (including cataplexy, hypnagogic hallucinations and sleep paralysis), this is the exception rather than the rule. Usually post-traumatic hypersomnia does not consist of cataplexy or REM-related abnormalities characteristic of narcolepsy. The most important point in making this diagnosis is the clear association with head trauma, i.e. that the sleepiness was clearly not observed before the trauma. Usually immediately after the trauma, the patients start to sleep for a longer duration during the night, experience naps and, despite these, may remain sleepy throughout the day. These symptoms may worsen over the short term (6–18 months after the trauma), and then experience some spontaneous improvement. Sometimes the diagnosis becomes complicated as the whole sleep–wake pattern changes because there are several case reports of development of circadian abnormalities following trauma. In these cases, the diagnosis of hypersomnia is rather difficult.

In the syndrome of post-traumatic hypersomnia, other signs of head trauma usually, although not necessarily, exist. These include headaches, impaired cognitive functions such as concentration and memory, and many experience frank neurological signs such as muscle hypotonia, changes in deep tendon reflexes, pathological reflexes, ataxia, etc. Further neurological evaluation is indicated in this syndrome, even if the initial trauma was mild and neurological investigation was not carried out at that time. This may include brain imaging (magnetic resonance imaging or MRI), full-montage EEG, and sometimes a SPECT (single photon emission computed tomography) or Doppler test of cerebral blood flow. It should be emphasized that this syndrome is different from the post-traumatic stress disorder that refers to a predominantly psychological trauma, and is usually manifested as insomnia rather than hypersomnia (and is discussed in Chapter 6). Furthermore, disorders of initiating and maintaining sleep are much more likely to complicate any given head trauma than the post-traumatic hypersomnia.

The mechanism of sleepiness following head trauma is not very well understood, although it is postulated that the brain regions responsible primarily for wakefulness are involved. These may include the lateral and/or posterior hypothalamus, basal forebrain, the posterior fossa and the pineal region. Involvement of these regions in other diseases such as hydrocephalus, ischaemia (cerebrovascular accident or CVA) or tumour may also result in hypersomnolence. The severity of the sleepiness seems to relate to the severity of the head trauma. Coma for 24 hours, head fracture and neurosurgical interventions were reported as predictors of more severe sleepiness. The head trauma in some cases may result in respiratory abnormalities as well, in which case it may be difficult to determine whether the sleepiness is primary or secondary. A second evaluation may be needed after treatment of the respiratory abnormality to distinguish between the two.

The natural history of post-traumatic hypersomnia is not very well established, although it may be expected that in the long run there will be spontaneous improvement. However, in the short term (up to 18 months after the trauma) it may worsen. Whenever a progressive course is observed, one should suspect another diagnosis such as primary CNS disease, e.g. hydrocephalus, epilepsy, subdural haematoma, tumour or chronic meningoencephalitis. Legal issues should also be considered because sometimes patients have secondary gain from being sleepy and may exaggerate their complaints.

There is no specific treatment and therapy should therefore be individualized. First-line treatment should deal with the underlying problem if possible (e.g. treat post-traumatic epilepsy or any neurological disorder that exists). Sleepiness resulting from antiepileptic medications should also be considered in the differential diagnosis. Symptomatic therapy may be similar to the treatment of IH and include improvement of sleep hygiene and the use of stimulant medications (see Table 24).

In summary, post-traumatic hypersomnia reflects sleepiness, which occurs up to 18 months after head trauma. To make this diagnosis, sleepiness needs to be objectively established, and a careful history is necessary to ensure the absence of hypersomnolence before the trauma.

chapter 7

Hypersomnia: summary and patient approach

As discussed elsewhere, a normal individual who gets adequate sleep should be able to maintain wakefulness during the day with little to no difficulty. When such an individual consistently falls asleep if not actively stimulated or in passive situations (watching television, reading, at the theatre, driving), this probably represents a clinical problem. It should, however, be distinguished from fatigue, which is seen in many medical and psychological disorders. People with true hypersomnolence, as opposed to fatigue, often fall asleep unintentionally. Tired people, on the other hand, complain about ‘exhaustion’ and ‘lack of energy’ rather than about falling asleep unintentionally. Minimal research, however, has been done on this ‘language of sleepiness’, and so much of what we know about this subject is based on clinical experience alone. When history cannot confidently help to distinguish fatigue from sleepiness, a Multiple Sleep Latency Test (MSLT) is indicated.

The most common cause of excessive sleepiness is obstructive sleep apnoea (OSA) (right-hand side of Figure 14). Thus, if a sleepy individual complains of loud snoring and witnessed apnoeas, polysomnography (PSG) is indicated and the most likely diagnosis is OSA. It should be noted, however, that other forms of sleep apnoea syndrome (SAS) may also exist (e.g. central sleep apnoea, Cheyne–Stokes respiration). If sleepiness exists without OSA, several potential aetiologies should be considered (Figure 14). These include other causes for sleep fragmentation, mainly periodic limb movement disorder (PLMD) (especially if the

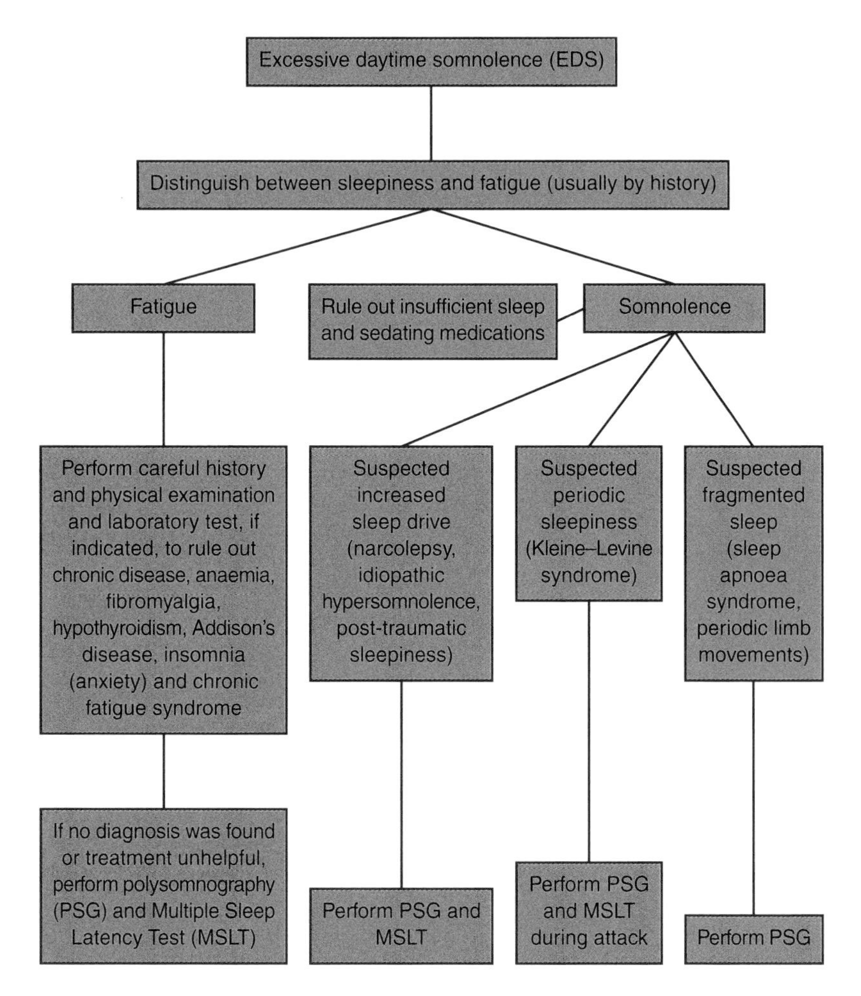

Figure 14 *Flow chart of the approach to the hypersomnolent/tired patient.*

patient complains of restless leg syndrome or RLS, or has been witnessed to 'kick' a lot during sleep), or primary sleepiness. The last may suggest narcolepsy if the patient has cataplexy, hypnagogic hallucinations, sleep paralysis or automatic behaviour in sleep.

A history of head trauma may put forward post-traumatic sleepiness (PTS), and true sleepiness without all the above can result from idiopathic hypersomnolence (IH). A periodic characteristic of the sleepiness with normal periods inbetween is suggestive of the Klein–Levine syndrome (KLS), especially if the hypersomnolent periods are accompanied by excessive eating and hypersexuality. When a patient is sleepy, some 'obvious' causes need to be ruled out, including inadequate sleep time (chronic insufficient sleep), hypnotic medication use and severe depression, which can usually be determined from the history.

Most people require at least 7 hours of sleep per night and often closer to 8. If the patient is sleeping less than this, total sleep time should be increased either before other diagnoses are considered or while other possibilities are being explored. Adequate daytime alertness after longer than usual sleep time supports insufficient sleep syndrome. If a patient is sleepy and being treated with medications that may cause sleepiness, the therapy should be re-evaluated and medications replaced or ceased if possible. Finally, if the history or MSLT suggests fatigue rather than sleepiness, several causes should be considered. First, almost every chronic illness can result in fatigue and exhaustion, including congestive heart failure, chronic anaemia, endocrine disorders (hypothyroidism, Addison's disease), collagen vascular disease (rheumatoid arthritis, systemic lupus erythematosus [SLE], temporal arthritis) and others (multiple sclerosis, multiple myeloma, any neoplastic disease, Parkinson's disease). Second, psychiatric disorders also frequently result in excessive fatigue (depression, anxiety). Finally, when a patient is fatigued with no notable reason, 'chronic fatigue syndrome' should be considered. As some of these diagnoses are not discussed elsewhere in this book, the following is a brief summary of them.

Fatigue

Hypothyroidism

The lack of, or insufficient secretion of, thyroid hormones results in hypometabolism and decreased caloric expenditure. As a result, many clinical features are associated with hypothyroidism, including sleepiness, lethargy, constipation, cold intolerance, muscle cramps, reduced motor activity and intellectual abilities, mild weight gain, dry and fragile hair, dry skin, hoarseness, etc. Some secondary disorders may develop such as OSA, hypercholesterolaemia and consequently ischaemic heart disease, megacolon or intestinal obstruction. In the sleep arena, hypothyroidism may be strongly associated with both fatigue and sleepiness. The decreased metabolic rate can cause the sensation of exhaustion, whereas the myxoedema, increased weight and secondary OSA can cause true hypersomnolence. Furthermore, the anaemia that is often seen in hypothyroid patients can also contribute to the fatigue.

Many of the classic features of hypothyroidism are associated with each other and with sleepiness, such as decreased intellectual function, altered mood, difficulties tolerating cold, etc. Thus, hypothyroidism should be considered in the evaluation of every tired and sleepy patient, especially in elderly people (the prevalence increases in this age group). Diagnosis is easily confirmed by a blood test of thyroid-stimulating hormone (TSH) and free thyroxine (T_4). Once diagnosed, treatment with levothyroxine is usually indicated (initially daily dose of 25 μg, and titrated up until a normal metabolic rate is sustained).

Addison's disease (hypoadrenalism)

Glucocorticoids, like thyroid hormones, are involved in the metabolism of proteins, carbohydrates, lipids and nucleic acids. They raise blood glucose (insulin antagonists), and modify fat and protein metabolism differently in various tissues. Adrenocortical hypofunction results in insufficient secretion of the adrenal steroid hormones. The clinical characteristics vary between patients, and may include some or all of the following: progressive fatigue, weakness, anorexia, nausea, vomiting, weight loss, cutaneous pigmentation, hypotension and potentially hypoglycaemia. With regard to sleep, hypoadrenalism has traditionally been associated with fatigue rather than sleepiness. However, hypoadrenalism may be a part of hypopituitarism, in which case true sleepiness may occur. The diagnosis is confirmed by the failure to increase plasma steroid levels (cortisol and 17-hydroxysteroids) upon administration of corticotrophin (ACTH test). Once diagnosed, hydrocortisone replacement therapy (and sometimes mineralocorticoids as well) is usually indicated.

Chronic fatigue syndrome

The chronic fatigue syndrome (CFS) is a not very well-defined multifactorial disorder with somatic and mental symptoms. The clinical picture varies among patients and may include weakness, fatigue, headaches, nausea, vertigo, cold intolerance, low-grade fever or mild hypothermia, hypotension, irregular pulse rate, irritable bowel, recurrent sore throat, arthralgias, myalgias, muscle cramps and sleep disorders. Mental changes are also common (either a cause or an effect) and include anxiety, depression, personality changes, memory and cognitive impairment and emotional instability. It may begin as a flu-like disease (frequently after infectious mononucleosis) and persist into a chronic phase (at least 6 months for diagnosis) with severe effects on daily life. The most common complaint is muscle weakness and general exhaustion, physical and mental, with an inability to maintain normal living. The syndrome probably consists of several different pathophysiological processes, and so the symptoms vary. Nevertheless, typically the patient's activity is dramatically reduced, with persistent or relapsing fatigue, and no alleviation by bed-rest or sleep. The age of onset is usually early adulthood (age 20–40), and women are affected more frequently. The natural history is not known, although most patients spontaneously recover after 1–6 years. In some patients the symptoms resemble other known illnesses such as multiple sclerosis, fibromyalgia, post-polio syndrome, hepatitis or autoimmune diseases, such as SLE. Physical examination may reveal lymphadenopathy with tenderness, non-exudative pharyngitis, muscle or joint tenderness, and mental changes.

As there is no pathognomonic diagnostic test, making the diagnosis is somewhat difficult. Some laboratory tests that have been reported in this syndrome include leukocytosis, leukopenia, lymphocytosis, anaemia, increased sedimentation rate and mild-to-moderate transaminase elevation. From the standpoint of sleep, this syndrome is clearly a problem of fatigue rather than sleepiness. A nocturnal sleep study may reveal increased sleep latency, difficulties maintaining sleep and decreased sleep efficiency. The EEG frequently has the α–δ sleep pattern, with α intrusion during the entire recording. Despite the patient's complaint of fatigue and even sleepiness, the MSLT is normal and typically does not demonstrate decreased sleep latency (i.e. excessive sleepiness). As the aetiology is unknown, and the diagnosis is difficult, there is no single therapeutic approach. Treatment should be individualized and may include medications (pain-killers, antidepressants, anxiolytics, hypnotics), behavioural therapy (psychotherapy, exercise, supporting groups, biofeedback), and other treatments such as changing diet (especially adding vitamins and essential fatty acids) or antiviral treatment (amantadine, aciclovir or interferon).

chapter 8

Insomnia

What is insomnia?

What is insomnia but the mad obstinacy of our mind in manufacturing thoughts and trains of reasoning, syllogisms and definitions of its own, refusing to abdicate in favor of that divine stupidity of closed eyes, or the wise folly of dreams? The man who cannot sleep . . . refuses more or less consciously to entrust himself to the flow of things.

Marguerite Yourcenar in *Memoirs of Hadrian*.
Grace Frick (trans.): NY: Farrar, Straus and Giroux, 1954.

Suffering from insomnia: a physician's account

Soon I ceased to sleep altogether, an attack of insomnia set in, so terrible that it nearly made me go off my head. Insomnia does not kill its man unless he kills himself – sleeplessness is the most common cause of suicide. But it kills his *joie de vivre*, it saps his strength, it sucks the blood from his brain and from his heart as a vampire. It makes him remember during the night what he was meant to forget in blissful sleep. It makes him forget during the day what he meant to remember . . . Voltaire was right when he placed sleep in the same level as hope.

Axel Munthe, physician, who suffered from life-long
insomnia, and author of *The Story of San Michele*.
London: John Murray, 1975.

Although a common clinical problem, there has been minimal research emphasis on the subject of insomnia. Therefore, the data about epidemiology, underlying mechanisms and therapy are all somewhat incomplete. In fact, we lack reliable data on the burden of disease, the appropriate pharmacological targets and the neurobiological basis of insomnia.

The available estimates suggest that roughly 20–35% of the general population has had difficulty sleeping in the previous year. Insomnia appears to be more common among women and among those of increasing age. Over 50% of elderly patients may complain of difficulties with nocturnal sleep. These figures may be even higher among hospitalized or institutionalized patients. This chapter presents the data available about the research into and the clinical aspects of insomnia.

Definition and diagnosis

The definition of insomnia is the perception of inadequate quantity or quality of sleep with associated daytime consequences. The definition is from the patient's perspective and therefore diagnostic testing is not generally required because history alone is sufficient to establish the diagnosis. There are two general approaches to the classification of insomnia based on either 'lumpers' or 'splitters'. Many clinicians feel that the various different types of insomnia have substantial overlap (see Table 28) and that the creation of artificial classification systems does not change clinical management. Others argue that insomnia patients may have variable complaints depending on the specific type of insomnia that they have and that classifying them may help guide therapy. We discuss each entity as distinct, but recognize that many patients have features of several forms of insomnia.

The four most common complaints of all forms of insomnia are difficulties falling asleep, frequent awakenings from sleep, difficulties falling back to sleep after nocturnal awakenings and spontaneous early morning awakening. By definition, as mentioned above, these complaints must be associated with daytime symptoms (i.e. fatigue, impaired concentration or memory, etc.), i.e. an individual who sleeps only 5 hours per night and cannot sleep more (either as a result of delayed falling asleep or secondary to early morning awakening) will not be diagnosed as insomniac if there is no daytime fatigue or impairment of daytime function. As mentioned in Chapter 2, most adults need 8–9 hours of sleep per night but some people habitually sleep for short periods of time (less than 6 hours per night) and are still able to function at high levels with no daytime complaints. Such people are considered 'physiologically short sleepers' and represent one extreme of the bell-shaped curve of sleep requirements in the general population. Again, by definition, these individuals are not insomniacs and in our experience, they are somewhat rare, in as much as many so-called 'short sleepers' have previously unrecognized daytime consequences.

Short-/long-term insomnia

An artificial cut-off of 3 weeks has been assigned as the distinction between acute and chronic insomnia. Acute insomnia is an extremely common complaint with most individuals experiencing some symptoms of insomnia on occasion throughout their lives. The majority of such cases probably never come to clinical fruition. Occasionally, for example, during acute stress such as a family death, some loss of sleep can be considered quite normal. However, if this is of sufficient concern to the afflicted individual, a brief course of a short-acting hypnotic is a reasonable treatment strategy (see later section on treatment). Chronic insomnia develops in those individuals with acute insomnia who have a particular predisposition, based on either genetic or environmental factors. Some sources also use the term 'transient insomnia', referring to difficulty with sleeping for less than 1 week. As can be derived from its name, short-term insomnia generally resolves and is usually not associated with major sequelae or complications. On the other hand, if it persists, long-term insomnia is associated with substantial consequences and potentially severe impairment in quality of life, as well as physical and mental condition. People with chronic insomnia are vulnerable to

Table 28 Classification of chronic insomnia (frequently there is an overlap between diagnoses)

	Psychophysiological insomnia	*Idiopathic insomnia*	*Sleep state misperception*
Prevalence (approximate) (%)	2–5	0.5	0.5
Age of onset (years)	20–40	Childhood	Any
Sex	Women > men	Women > men	Women > men
PSG findings	Frequently reversed first-night effect	Insomnia (long SL, low SE)	Normal sleep pattern
Main treatment approach (in addition to sleep hygiene)	Cognitive–behavioural, relaxation, hypnotics	Supportive	Reassurance/ Supportive

PSG, polysomnography; SL, sleep latency; SE, sleep efficiency.

fatigue-related injuries and road traffic accidents. They are more likely to complain of poor stamina for completing routine tasks and deficits in concentration. If patients with chronic insomnia were not nervous and irritable before the insomnia, they will become so as a result of it. They are also likely to become sad and depressed. As a consequence of these changes in the physical and mental condition of insomnia patients, their performance at work and home deteriorates, and they are susceptible to loss of work or divorce. People with insomnia utilize medical care more than twice as much as their matched controls who do not have insomnia.

Psychophysiological insomnia

Psychophysiological insomnia is one of the more common aetiologies of chronic insomnia that is a clinical diagnosis. Typically, such patients initially experience some acute stress, which leads to insomnia; this would be transient in most individuals. In certain predisposed individuals, however, the acute insomnia leads to substantial concern and distress about their inability to sleep. The result is a vicious cycle of poor sleep, leading to further anxiety about insomnia, which contributes further to the problem. These patients are frequently also tense and anxious, but they become so focused on their sleep disorder that they tend to minimize other mental concerns. It typically occurs at young adulthood (ages 20–40) and is substantially more common in women than in men. As stated, the diagnosis is usually made by history alone. However, if polysomnography (PSG) is performed, they may demonstrate insomniac features (prolonged sleep latency, fragmented sleep, α intrusion into the EEG in all stages of sleep, early morning awakening), but frequently demonstrate the opposite, i.e. reversed first night effect. Normally individuals tend to sleep worse in their first night in the laboratory (a term referred to 'first night effect'). Patients with psychophysiological insomnia frequently sleep better in the laboratory than in their home, probably secondary to breaking this vicious cycle by changing the sleep environment.

In addition to general therapeutic measures for insomnia, the treatment involves interruption of the cycle by reassurance and in some cases cognitive–behavioural therapy. Stimulus control therapy is targeted at controlling the stimuli (the bedroom and bedtime ritual) that became aversive and cause the problem. Removing the alarm clock from the bedroom may be particular beneficial for these individuals as the knowledge of time spent awake can contribute greatly to anxiety and further insomnia. The other characteristic feature of these patients is the history of improved sleep when in a foreign environment. Thus, changing the sleep environment may also be beneficial in patients with psychophysiological insomnia. The foreign environment alleviates some of the cues to which the patient has become conditioned, and thus relieves the associated anxiety.

Idiopathic insomnia

As the name would imply, idiopathic insomnia is a diagnosis of exclusion. Typically these individuals experience lifelong symptoms of insomnia and are generally refractory to therapy. Therefore, the focus on treatment, in addition to general therapeutic measures for insomnia, should include frank discussions with patients about the chronicity of the disease. Helping patients to accept their disease and enhancing coping skills are two goals for patients with idiopathic insomnia

> 'I must not forget that I never slept a wink.' Never sleeping a wink was her great claim to distinction, and one admitted and respected in our household vocabulary; . . . during the day, when my aunt wished to take a nap, we used to say just that she wished to 'be quiet' or 'to rest'; and in the conversation she so far forgot herself as to say 'What woke me up?' or 'I dreamt that,' she would blush and at once correct herself.
>
> Marcel Proust on his insomniac aunt, in *Remembrance of Things Past*. CK Scott Moncrieff and Terence Kilmartin (trans.) Swann's Way, Chatto, 1929.

Sleep state misperception

Many patients with chronic insomnia have poor perception of the total amount of time spent asleep. Thus a number of patients who present to the physician describing only 3–4 hours of sleep per night will in fact have 6–7 hours of sleep when sleep is objectively measured. This phenomenon of sleep state misperception can be present in patients with any of the listed aetiologies of chronic insomnia. As insomnia is a subjective complaint, the focus in these patients should not be in 'disproving' their symptoms. Instead, treatment should be conducted as for other aetiologies of insomnia. Objective documentation of total sleep time can be reassuring for some patients. In such individuals, objective testing can be used to alleviate anxiety about chronic insomnia. However, as stated, some insomnia patients will demonstrate improved sleep efficiency during laboratory PSG. Thus, the use of objective testing should be individualized.

Inadequate sleep hygiene

Poor sleep hygiene is a frequent contributor to inadequate total sleep time among patients who have insomnia for other reasons. Thus, many individuals may practise poor sleep hygiene, but in the absence of a predisposing condition may have no demonstrable sleep abnormalities. However, among most patients who present to the healthcare provider with complaints related to sleep, poor sleep hygiene is frequently an issue.

Factors that may contribute to chronic insomnia in these individuals may be classified into those resulting in increased nocturnal alertness and those that interfere with sleep continuity. Arousing factors include excessive caffeine, frequent naps, vigorous exercise close to bedtime and stressful/exciting work at night. Factors that disturb sleep continuity consist of falling asleep with the TV or radio on, alcoholic drinks (resulting in the need to urinate at night), environmental factors (noise, uncomfortable ambient temperature, uncomfortable bed, snoring/

moving bed partner, light) and excessive time in bed. Excessive time in bed and frequent naps are special problem in elderly people and in unemployed or institutionalized individuals. People with no work or daily obligations frequently find themselves asleep during the day, with a subsequent inability to fall asleep at night. It is very important to understand that the physiology of sleep does not allow accumulation of sleep (generating a bank of sleep), i.e. when the sleep need is low, an individual usually is unable to sleep. This is the logical basis for the 'sleep restriction' approach. By restricting time in bed and eliminating diurnal sleep, the drive to sleep is increased and, with the opening of the 'sleep gate' in the evening or early night, the individual can fall asleep more easily. As stated in the treatment section below, many patients will benefit from a simple review of the sleep hygiene recommendations listed in Table 32.

Restless leg syndrome

The restless leg syndrome (RLS) is a common disorder which is generally diagnosed clinically. Although minimal work has been carried out on the neurobiology of RLS, the available evidence points to abnormalities in the dopamine (D_3) receptors in the mesolimbic system. Although it may coexist with periodic limb movement disorder (PLMD), these entities are discussed separately because they may present quite differently. Although RLS commonly presents with insomnia and is discussed here, PLMD usually presents as fragmentation of sleep leading to excessive daytime sleepiness and is discussed in Chapter 5.

The true prevalence of RLS is unclear because most cases remain undiagnosed. Some questionnaire-based surveys suggest that over 10% of the general North American population may have symptoms consistent with this disorder. However, a more realistic estimate of prevalence is roughly 5% of the general population. As a result of lack of awareness of this disorder on the part of patients, as well as healthcare providers, the median time from onset of symptoms to diagnosis is over 15 years in some series.

Restless leg syndrome is generally a clinical diagnosis based on a constellation of four features (Table 29). First, patients have sensory complaints that are referable to the lower extremities. These complaints may be 'pain', although they are more commonly described as 'achy' or 'creepy crawly' symptoms. Second, motor complaints are generally seen in RLS patients. The characteristic description is one of 'restlessness' or the 'need to pace' or the 'need to get up and walk around'. Third, the motor and sensory symptoms are typically worse at rest. Many patients with an active lifestyle are unaware of the symptoms unless they are sedentary (e.g. eating a meal). Fourth and finally, these complaints are usually worse at night. The classic description from insomnia patients is an inability to sleep because of ongoing lower extremity discomfort or the need to get up and walk rather than lying in bed. Although studies are incomplete, the available data suggest that the pattern of RLS is circadian in nature. Without careful questioning about these four criteria, many patients will go undiagnosed.

There are a number of entities that have been associated with RLS (Table 30). Once a diagnosis of RLS has been made, these underlying causes should be considered. Iron deficiency anaemia is a common underlying cause, and should be excluded in all RLS patients. A full panel of iron indices (ferritin, transferrin saturation, mean corpuscular volume, haemoglobin) should be checked, because many of these patients do not have overt anaemia. Although the gold standard for the diagnosis of iron deficiency is a bone marrow biopsy, this is not a practical test to perform in this clinical setting. The mechanism underlying the RLS secondary to iron deficiency is thought to involve dopamine biosynthesis because iron is both a co-factor for synthetic enzymes

Table 29 Diagnostic criteria for restless leg syndrome

1	Sensory complaints in the lower extremities
2	Motor restlessness in the lower extremities
3	Worse at rest
4	Worse at night

(tyrosine hydroxylase) and involved in some dopaminergic receptors. Other entities that should be considered in the work-up for underlying causes of RLS should include selective serotonin reuptake inhibitors, tricyclic antidepressants, peripheral neuropathy, renal failure, rheumatoid arthritis and congestive heart failure. In the case of end-stage renal failure, RLS may be particularly important because it has been associated with increased mortality and may respond to erythropoietin therapy.

The treatment of RLS is based on the predominant symptom (Table 31). Although many of these patients have coexisting PLMD, in this section we focus on the awake symptoms described above. The first step in therapy is treatment of the underlying cause. Therefore, if any of the underlying causes are identified, the initial efforts should be directed at reversing these factors, if possible. Assuming that pharmacological therapy for the RLS is required, the mainstay of treatment is with dopaminergic medications. A number of different medications are available, although the most commonly used ones are L-dopa/carbidopa (Sinemet) and pramipexole (Mirapex). Although the former medication had been the usual first-line treatment for RLS, pramipexole is now emerging as the treatment of choice, based on recent randomized trials. The clinical experience with pramipexole has also been favourable, with little if any dose escalation on long-term follow-up. Side effects from this medication are minimal, although patients should be warned of rare reports of road traffic accidents resulting in Parkinson's disease patients who have received this medication from falling asleep while driving. If

Table 30 Underlying causes of restless leg syndrome

1	Iron deficiency anaemia
2	Selective serotonin reuptake inhibitors (SSRIs)
3	Tricyclic antidepressants (TCAs)
4	Rheumatoid arthritis
5	Peripheral neuropathy
6	Congestive heart failure
7	Renal failure

Table 31 Treatment of restless leg syndrome

Underlying cause
Dopaminergics:
  Sinemet (L-dopa/carbidopa)
  Mirapex (pramipexole)
Antiepileptics:
  Neurontin (gabapentin)
Opioids:
  propoxyphene
Iron supplements

L-dopa/carbidopa therapy is undertaken, the long-acting medication (Sinemet CR) is preferred because it is associated with improved efficacy and fewer symptoms as the medication wears off. Other medications that have some efficacy in the treatment of RLS include the antiepileptic medications (e.g. gabapentin) and the opioids. Although many clinicians are concerned about the potential for abuse of opioids, minimal dose escalation has been observed in long-term follow-up studies. Finally, for refractory cases, some consider supplemental iron, even for patients with no objective evidence of iron deficiency.

Insomnia associated with psychiatric disorders

Many patients with psychiatric disorders experience difficulties related to sleep. A common clinical problem is to distinguish the effects of medications from the effects of the underlying disorders. This distinction frequently requires careful history taking and review of medical records to establish the onset of symptoms in relation to specific medications. Occasionally, a diagnostic trial of medication withdrawal is required to determine the attributable effect of medication on symptoms. Such trials should be conducted in conjunction with strict supervision by treating psychiatrists. As a result of the nature of this patient population, many of the insomnia-related complaints go undiagnosed without careful questioning on the part of the healthcare provider.

Although not always part of the diagnostic criteria, insomnia and sleep disruption are characteristic features of a number of different psychiatric disorders. Specifically, patients with depression frequently experience early morning wakening. Although patients with mania frequently have very little sleep, they typically do not complain of difficulty sleeping and therefore do not have insomnia by the classic definition. Interestingly, sleep deprivation is frequently associated with mania, and therefore it has been proposed as a therapy for depression. Patients with schizophrenia and Alzheimer's disease may have day/night reversal for somewhat unclear reasons. In post-traumatic stress disorder (PTSD), sleep disturbances are incorporated in the definition, and are required for diagnosis, which includes re-experiencing symptoms (nightmares) and the hyperarousal state (difficulty initiating and maintaining sleep). Moreover, insomnia, restless sleep and trauma-related dreams are frequently the primary complaint of these patients.

Both generalized anxiety disorder and panic disorder are associated with disruption of sleep. Patients with both of these diagnoses frequently have associated insomnia. In particular some patients with panic disorder will have panic attacks, primarily in the middle of the night. These nocturnal panic attacks can be extremely frightening to the patient and the bed partner. They typically occur in stages 2 and 3 of sleep and must be distinguished from parasomnias and other disorders.

Depression is frequently complicated by difficulty sleeping, in particular early morning wakening. In approximately 30% of patients with major depression, the primary complaint is related to sleep (i.e. insomnia, hypersomnia or dream disorders), and it is not uncommon that the first physician who makes the diagnosis is a sleep physician rather than a psychiatrist. Of particular concern is the fact that insomnia in patients with depression is a predictor of suicide tendency. Several studies have suggested that patients with both depression and insomnia are particularly at risk of committing suicide. Thus, careful history taking is required in such patients to assess the potential risk for such behaviours. Although the diagnosis of depression is a clinical one, some patients mask their behaviours and the diagnosis is difficult to establish. A sleep study (PSG) is, in fact, one of the sole objective tools to suggest the diagnosis of depression. Depressed patients often demonstrate a short REM latency (30–50 min), increased REM sleep percentage (>30% of total sleep time) increased REM density (frequent and intense eye movements during REM sleep), and spontaneous early morning awakening. Moreover, follow-up sleep studies may help to determine the efficacy of treatment. Antidepressant medications reverse the effects of depression on sleep. The therapeutic decision should always consider the sleep pattern in a depressed patient. In patients whose primary sleep disorder is from the insomnia group, a sedating antidepressant should be started (such as amitriptyline, trazodone or doxepine), whereas in hypersomnolent patients less sedating or non-sedating medications should be preferred (e.g. fluoxetine, protriptyline, nortriptyline, mianserin).

Eating disorders

Sleep-related eating disorders are a clinical syndrome that usually consists of the combination of an eating disorder and a sleep disorder. Patients (usually young women) typically experience nocturnal partial awakenings (usually in the first third of the night), during which they eat voraciously. They may eat unusual combinations of food, or or inedible items that they usually do not eat while awake (e.g. inanimate objects such as books). In addition, they may leave a huge mess, after eating in a sloppy manner. For these reasons, some doctors believe this is primarily a parasomnia, and classify it as a 'disorder of arousal'. However, in contrast to the disorders of arousal, patients with the sleep-related eating disorder not uncommonly suffer from psychiatric disorders such as anorexia nervosa, bulimia nervosa, binge eating disorder, affective disorder, generalized anxiety or PTSD. In addition, these patients, unlike 'simple sleep walkers', respond quite favourably to dopaminergic agents. However, many of these patients do not demonstrate any psychiatric disorder, and instead have a primary sleep disorder such as sleep walking, RLS, PLM or obstructive sleep apnoea (OSA). Treatment for sleep-related nocturnal eating is recommended and is frequently successful in reducing weight and improving sleep.

Cognitive–behavioural therapy, hypnosis and biofeedback are usually ineffective. Dopaminergic agents alone or in combination with opioids, SSRIs or clonazepam are recommended.

Post-traumatic stress disorder

Post-traumatic stress disorder is an increasingly recognized diagnosis which is used to describe individuals who suffer from neuropsychological problems experienced after a psychologically traumatic event. The most frequent sleep-related complaints of these patients are difficulties falling asleep, frequent awakenings from sleep (with further difficulties falling back to sleep), shorter sleep duration, restless sleep, daytime fatigue and especially flashbacks during sleep (nightmares, anxiety dreams). Polysomnographic studies of PTSD patients' sleep architecture have produced conflicting results. PTSD patients tend to sleep only slightly worse than controls. In many studies, differences in PSG measures between PTSD patients and controls were negligible or not statistically significant. Nevertheless, changes in REM sleep and dreaming may occur. Both shortening and elongation of REM latency, and lower and higher REM percentages, have been reported in PTSD, and in fact the extremely high variability of these measures might be relatively specific for this disorder. REM density is increased and phasic events during REM sleep (e.g. muscle twitches) are elevated. Dream recall is lower in chronic PTSD patients compared with normal controls but, when they do recall dreams, these are more hostile and threatening. There is no specific treatment for PTSD-related sleep disorders. Therapy may consist of psychotherapy, antidepressants, hypnotics and other psychotropic medications, and should be individualized for each patient depending on the dominance of the symptoms with which he or she presents.

Insomnia associated with medical disorders

Complaints about difficulties with sleep are exceedingly common among medical patients. Difficulties with sleep may be related to pain, shortness of breath, medication effects or specific disorders. Regardless of the mechanism, the prevalence of these complaints among this patient population is high. Therefore, we recommend at least one question about sleep in the review of systems that is conducted during the initial history taking and physical examination. In some cases, treatment of the underlying medical disorder will alleviate the sleep-related symptoms. However, in many cases, patients perceive poor sleep as a huge problem, requiring specific attention in addition to their other medical issues.

Chronic pain (rheumatoid arthritis, headache, cancer)

Particularly among medical patients, issues of chronic pain can contribute to difficulties with sleeping. In some cases, pain can lead to inability to fall asleep (sleep initiation insomnia), whereas in others chronic pain can be associated with repeated or prolonged arousal (sleep maintenance insomnia). Frequently, patients taking chronic analgesics will experience worsening of their pain after the effects of these medications wear off. Thus, such patients experience early morning wakening unless given adequately dosed, long-acting, analgesic medications. Sleep disruption may in fact have clinical value in assessing a patient with chronic pain, e.g. patients with headaches (tension headaches or migraines) often suffer from pain while awake, but may sleep well. This is generally an indication of a relatively mild pain. Patients who wake up from sleep with pain probably suffer from a worse attack of headaches, and in children awakenings from sleep with headaches are one of the indications for a computed tomography (CT) of the head. Patients with chronic nocturnal awakenings caused by headaches, similar to other chronic pain syndromes, may develop chronic insomnia with the associated further consequences discussed above.

For certain diagnoses, morning symptoms are particularly prevalent, e.g. although the predictive value is variable, morning headache has been associated with obstructive sleep apnoea syndrome in some series. Similarly, morning stiffness is one of the diagnosed criteria for rheumatoid arthritis. Finally some patients such as those with fibromyalgia can experience insomnia caused by non-restorative sleep with substantial α intrusion seen in the EEG. Chronic pain is one entity that usually requires specific therapy to alleviate insomnia rather than non-specific hypnotic medications.

For many years, it has been well known among oncologists and their patients that patients with cancer suffer from insomnia. This can result from any combination of a variety of factors, such as the direct effect of disease on sleep generation, the effect of disease mediated by immune messengers (e.g. certain cytokines), effects of chronic pain, nausea, vomiting, mental factors such as anxiety or depression, or side effects of chemotherapy or steroids. Regardless of the mechanism, insomnia very frequently complicates problems for oncology patients and presents a great challenge for the treating physician. It is well documented that hypnotics are the most frequently prescribed psychotropic medication in cancer patients. Whether other treatments may be effective is unknown at this time, because only limited research has targeted this issue. However, some data suggest that cognitive–behavioural and relaxation therapy may be beneficial. Patients with cancer should be prepared for the possibility that sleep will be impaired, and just discussing this with them may be helpful. Finally, preliminary data suggest that melatonin may be of value.

Breathing disorders (asthma, apnoea, cystic fibrosis)

Shortness of breath in the middle of the night can be a distressing complaint for afflicted individuals. In some cases, waking up gasping for breath can be sufficiently frightening to patients that they may be unable to sleep for the remainder of the night. Thus, the priorities should include work-up for aetiology of shortness of breath, as well as reassurance if appropriate.

A great deal of information can be gained about the aetiology of dyspnoea at night from the history alone (see Table 15). Although orthopnoea is commonly associated with congestive heart failure, the presence of immediate orthopnoea (i.e. short latency) should direct a search towards neuromuscular weakness, specifically diaphragmatic paralysis. This can be assessed using diaphragmatic fluoroscopy ('sniff test'), diaphragm ultrasonography or direct measurement of transdiaphragmatic pressure (oesophageal and gastric balloon). In patients with

Cheyne–Stokes respiration, some history of congestive heart failure, myocardial infarction and occasionally neurological disease is usually present. Patients with congestive heart failure who experience paroxysmal nocturnal dyspnoea generally do so during the hyperpnoeic phase of Cheyne–Stokes breathing. Patients with OSA commonly present with associated snoring and obesity. Although OSA patients characteristically present with excessive daytime sleepiness, there is a subgroup of these patients who present with insomnia, classically a sleep maintenance insomnia from recurrent arousals. Patients with central sleep apnoea (CSA), on the other hand, are more likely to present with a complaint of insomnia rather than daytime hypersomnolence. In this disorder, arousals from sleep (for any reason) are associated with temporary hyperventilation (for a few breaths) resulting in hypocapnia and subsequently apnoea, and this cycling may continue throughout the night. In some clinical circumstances, it may be unclear whether central apnoeas are contributing to insomnia or, conversely, whether insomnia is contributing to central apnoeas. In these instances, the use of sedative/hypnotic medications is frequently effective in eliminating these sleep transitions and the associated insomnia and breathing instability.

In patients with asthma, nocturnal awakenings should alert the clinician to potential trouble. The awakenings in nocturnal asthma are characteristically around 4 am, after daytime medications have worn off and sympathovagal balance favours bronchoconstriction. Nocturnal asthma symptoms are a marker of poor asthma control and should trigger more aggressive anti-inflammatory therapy. Of particular concern are data that suggest increased risk of status asthmaticus among those with frequent nocturnal symptoms. Other diseases that can contribute to shortness of breath at night are gastro-oesophageal reflux and coronary ischaemia. Finally, depression can present with early morning awakening and can mimic some of these respiratory disorders.

The treatment of insomnia caused by nocturnal shortness of breath is directed at the underlying cause. Treatment of OSA with nasal continuous positive airway pressure (CPAP) commonly leads to good sleep consolidation. Treatment of Cheyne–Stokes respiration by optimizing therapy of congestive heart failure (afterload reduction, diuresis) and/or

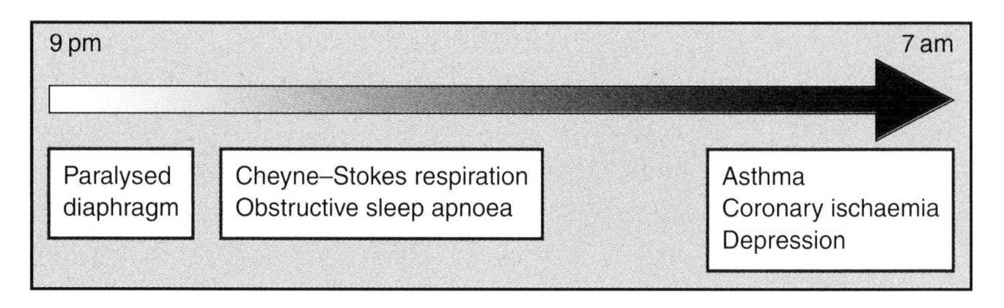

Figure 15 *Typical timing of insomnia associated with respiratory disorders.*

nasal CPAP also can improve sleep quality. As stated, treatment of nocturnal asthma includes inhaled glucocorticoids and possibly long-acting β_2-adrenoceptor agonists (e.g. salmeterol) and leukotriene-modifying medications (e.g. zafirlukast). Finally, treatment of coronary ischaemia typically involves β blockade and long-acting nitrates.

Another consideration for the work-up for insomnia in pulmonary patients is related to specific medications, e.g. β_2-adrenoceptor agonists, theophylline and systemic glucocorticoids may all contribute to difficulty with sleeping. Thus, in some cases, therapy may include withdrawal or substitution of culprit medications.

Movement disorders (Parkinson's disease, dystonia)

Parkinson's disease is thought to involve dopamine deficiency in the substantia nigra of the basal ganglia. Parkinson's disease has been associated with multiple different sleep disorders including OSA and CSA, insomnia (anxiety and depression), periodic limb movements, REM behavioural disorder, dementia and medication effects. Thus, quite a number of Parkinson's disease patients will have some form of sleep disorder if questioned carefully. For some of these patients, their sleep abnormalities are among their most distressing symptoms; thus, careful attention must be paid to this possibility. Although most of these sleep abnormalities are discussed elsewhere in this book, some issues in Parkinson's disease deserve specific emphasis.

In many cases, there is a diagnostic dilemma as to whether the patient's symptoms are from the Parkinson's disease itself or medication related. Also, in some instances, medication effects may be unpredictable, e.g. low doses of dopaminergic drugs may promote sleep, whereas higher doses may increase sleep-onset latency. Along these lines, high doses of dopaminergics may occasionally impair sleep in the first half of the night and promote better sleep in the second half of the night. Thus, a very careful history must be obtained by the treating clinician. In addition, diagnostic manoeuvres must be carefully monitored because they may worsen symptoms if the wrong aetiology is being treated.

Another potential source of diagnostic uncertainty in Parkinson's patients is that of nightmares. Although these patients are well known to be at increased risk of REM behavioural disorder (RBD), dopaminergic medications have been associated with severe nightmares. In fact, up to 30% of patients on dopaminergic medications will report vivid dreams, nightmares and night terrors. Particularly when treating patients with cognitive impairment, the distinction between these two entities (RBD and medication side effect) may be quite challenging. Clearly, the treatment of these entities is also very different (clonazepam for RDB and adjustment of medications for dopaminergic-induced nightmares). Thus treatment of the Parkinson's disease patient is frequently difficult, often requiring diagnostic trials of therapy and close long-term follow-up.

Nocturnal paroxysmal dystonia (NPD) is another movement disorder that can frequently mimic frontal lobe epilepsy and occasionally PLMD. There is in fact some controversy about whether NPD represents a form of temporal lobe epilepsy, because there are scattered reports of NPD responding to ablation of brain lesions (cortical dysplasia). However, NPD does not appear to respond to anticonvulsants in most cases. NPD typically occurs during NREM sleep and each episode lasts for several minutes (although some subclassify these into short and long attacks). The motor attacks are frequently complex behaviours with associated dyskinetic or ballistic movements. As there have been these reports of associated brain lesions, a careful neurological evaluation is recommended.

Neurological disorders

Although rare, fatal familial insomnia (FFI) is a frequently discussed entity because of its unique clinical features. FFI is a rare inherited prion disease which has been reported to occur in a large family cohort in Italy. Reports remote from this family have been exceedingly rare. The disease is characterized by the subacute progression of intractable insomnia up to a total absence of sleep, and is universally fatal. The deterioration period lasts several months and is associated, apart from the insomnia, with other autonomic, cerebellar and pyramidal manifestations as well with dementia. There are no known treatments for this disease, and patients die within several months of diagnosis.

Sleep disruption with epilepsy is a common clinical problem. Some sources estimate that up to one-third of people with epilepsy have seizures exclusively at night. Therefore, the diagnosis may be missed unless considered specifically. Furthermore, the usual EEG leads frequently miss seizure activity during routine PSG. Therefore, if the clinical suspicion for nocturnal seizures is high, an extended EEG montage should be requested during sleep recording. Treatment should be directed as for other forms of epilepsy, with antiepileptic medications and possibly surgical therapy.

Alzheimer's disease and other forms of dementia are frequently characterized by disruption of sleep. In many cases, patients with dementia have a loss of the day–night cycle and appear to have abnormalities in circadian rhythms. Some speculate that degeneration of the suprachiasmatic nucleus (the circadian pacemaker) may lead to these clinical phenomena. Sedative/hypnotic medications must be used cautiously in this patient population because of increased risk of falls and adverse drug events. 'Sundowning' is another common clinical problem in these patients because they commonly become more confused in the night. Medications such as clozapine or olanzapine may have some utility in this regard.

Circadian rhythm abnormalities (ASPS, DSPS, jet lag, shift work)

Circadian rhythm abnormalities are a frequent cause of sleep disruption. Advanced sleep phase syndrome (ASPS) classically occurs in older patients who habitually go to sleep early and wake up early. Conversely, delayed sleep phase syndrome (DPSP) patients are often teenagers who habitually go to sleep late and wake up late. We reserve these definitions for individuals who find these sleep patterns distressing, rather than those who choose their sleep schedule to fit lifestyle/behavioural factors. There is ongoing controversy about the aetiology of ASPS and DSPS, but they probably involve both genetic and environmental factors. The treatment of these disorders is an attempt to reset the circadian clock to the desired position. In the case of DSPS, this can be done with the use of melatonin therapy before sleep onset, which will serve to move the circadian clock progressively earlier. In addition, light exposure in the morning (after the nadir temperature), and the avoidance of light at night can both help to move the circadian clock earlier. Conversely, with ASPS, the treatment involves bright light exposure at night to shift the circadian clock later, and the avoidance of bright light in the morning analogous to DSPS.

Jet lag is an increasingly common clinical problem with the increases in long distance flights that have occurred in recent times. There are a number of factors that contribute to this problem, including a discrepancy between the circadian clock and the local time of day, the frequent naps that occur on airplanes, the intake of alcohol and caffeine, and the variable exposure to light and dark on the airplane, among others. Depending on the direction of travel, the treatment is quite different. In the case of an individual who is travelling from west to east, the administration of melatonin can be used to shift the circadian clock to avoid symptoms of jet lag. It should be given within 1–2 days before flying, at 7 pm on the target location time. It is reported to alleviate symptoms of jet lag in up to 50% of those who took it, and may shorten the habituation time from an average of 3–5 days to 2–3 days. In the case of east-to-west travel, the primary therapies involve education and the avoidance of sleep at intermittent or unscheduled times. We should note, however, that there is not much information about the long-term effects of melatonin and therefore it should be used with great caution.

Shift work is also increasingly common as a result of the demands placed by modern society. Although some individuals adapt well to variable schedules, others have substantial difficulty and suffer from so-called 'shift work insomnia'. These individuals have difficulty sleeping during the day after having worked during the night. The reason for this abnormality is unclear. On average, many shift workers sleep less in a 24-h period than individuals who sleep at conventional times. The optimal treatment of these individuals is unclear, but in general minimizing the number of nightshifts appears to be helpful. Others suggested that prolonged periods of consecutive nightshifts might be beneficial by allowing a better adaptation of the circadian system. A different approach is careful selection of shiftwork candidates who have no sleep disturbances and can easily adapt to an inversion of their sleep cycle.

> 'Hold him there, and take him away, for I'll make him sleep there tonight out of the air.'
>
> 'By God' said the lad, 'your worship can no more make me sleep in prison than make me king!'
>
> 'Well, why can't I make you sleep in prison?' asked Sancho.
>
> 'Now, my Lord Governor,' answered the youth, 'suppose your worship orders me to be taken to prison, and has me loaded with fetters and chains there and put in a cell, laying the jailer under heavy penalties to carry out your orders, and not let me out; all the same if I don't wish to sleep, and stay awake all night without closing an eyelid, will your worship with all your power be able to make me sleep if I don't choose to?'
>
> Miguel de Cervantes, *The Adventures of Don Quixote.*
> Samuel Putnam (trans.) NY: Viking, 1945.

Treatment

Apart from the specific therapies discussed above, minimal data are currently available on the optimal treatment of patients with insomnia.

However, evolving data suggest that inadequate nocturnal sleep may be associated with increased mortality (especially cardiovascular death) but these data are controversial. At the present time, it is unclear whether volitional (or lifestyle-driven) sleep restriction and insomnia have the same impact from the standpoint of health effects. As this is such a common clinical problem, however, a fair amount of empirical evidence and bedside observation has been made. Much of the therapy that is provided for patients with insomnia is therefore based on the 'art of medicine' rather than hard science or randomized controlled trials. Patient preference is also a major factor in choosing optimal treatment of insomnia. Many simple or 'commonsense' interventions are commonly overlooked, such as stopping caffeine intake or withdrawing culprit medications such as theophylline, glucocorticoids or selective serotonin reuptake inhibitors.

Behavioural/sleep hygiene, relaxation techniques, exercise

Despite incomplete data, treatment of insomnia patients is frequently effective with the use of rather simple modifications in sleep behaviour (see Table 32). These measures can be implemented for patients with any aetiology of insomnia, but are most helpful for those with poor sleep hygiene and for psychophysiological insomnias. Other therapeutic approaches include stimulus control (specific to psychophysiological insomnia), cognitive–behavioural psychotherapy and relaxation (by biofeedback, hypnosis, meditation, etc.), with or without hypnotic medications at least initially.

One recent randomized trial was published comparing cognitive–behavioural therapy with relaxation therapy and with placebo for the treatment of chronic primary (idiopathic) insomnia. The trial reported important improvements in WASO (wake after sleep onset) with cognitive–behavioural therapy, but only minor improvements with relaxation therapy and with placebo. Although far from definitive, the trial definitely supported the use of cognitive–behavioural therapy in the treatment of idiopathic insomnia.

Exercise is another treatment that is frequently employed in the treatment of insomnia. Although the treatment effect has not been subjected

Table 32 Sleep hygiene recommendations

1	Do not spend too much time in bed. Limit the time you spend in bed to sleeping. If you have woken up, get out of bed. Go back to bed only when you are ready to sleep.
2	Do not try to force yourself to sleep. The more you try to fall asleep, the more your arousal level will increase and falling asleep will become more difficult.
3	Remove the clock in your bedroom; its ticking and luminous dial can easily prevent you from falling asleep.
4	Avoid physical activity in the late evening hours. Exercise should be done at least 2 hours before going to bed.
5	Avoid drinking coffee and alcohol and smoking before going to bed.
6	Do not eat a heavy meal before going to bed.
7	Do not drink any beverages excessively before going to bed.
8	Go to sleep and wake up at regular hours. A routine in bedtime and waking-up hours is of great importance.
9	Do not sleep during the day.
10	Make sure that your sleep environment is as comfortable as possible (i.e. with respect to temperature, noise, light, etc.).

to randomized trials, our clinical experience with properly timed exercise has shown substantial improvements in chronic insomnia. If exercise takes place immediately before sleep, however, it may contribute to further difficulty in sleeping. The purported mechanism of this worsening is a sustained elevation in body temperature, which occurs after exercise. On the other hand, if exercise occurs 5 or more hours before sleep time, the latency to the onset of sleep is frequently reduced. Therefore, although the timing of exercise must be individualized, it is a reasonable treatment strategy for many chronic insomnia patients.

Sleep restriction is another commonly used treatment for insomnia. Many insomnia patients spend hours in bed while awake, which can further worsen conditioned insomnia. The concept underlying sleep restriction is gradually to improve the patient's sleep efficiency by limiting time spent in bed. Once adequate sleep efficiency has been obtained, the time spent in bed is gradually increased. Thus, the patient is not given the opportunity to spend prolonged periods of wakefulness in bed. During sleep restriction, patients who sleep poorly will develop progressive sleep deprivation and thus sleep better during the subsequent night. Over time, the patient 'learns' to sleep well and breaks the vicious cycle of anxiety and insomnia.

Benzodiazepines

Benzodiazepines are extremely commonly prescribed medications for the problem of insomnia. They are extremely effective hypnotics, with excellent data supporting their short-term use for symptomatic treatment of insomnia. However, there are minimal data for their use beyond 1 week of treatment. Although numerous different agents are available from this class of medication, they are clinically quite similar, with the exception of differences in half-life. For patients who have primarily sleep initiation insomnia, a very short-acting medication may be appropriate. Similarly, some of the ultra-short-acting medications may be useful for patients who require hypnotic medication in the middle of the night after a prolonged awakening. However, for patients with frequent awakenings throughout the night (sleep maintenance insomnia), a longer-acting medication may be preferable. Table 33 presents some of the commonly prescribed hypnotics, along with their dosage and half-life in the serum. Also, patient side effects may help guide the choice of medication, e.g. a patient who experiences a prolonged 'hang-over' in the morning after a particular medication would probably benefit from a shorter-acting one.

Patients who are given prescriptions for benzodiazepines should have both the risks and benefits discussed with them. Although these medications are relatively safe, there is some potential for abuse. Many patients who stop taking benzodiazepines will actually experience a rebound worsening of their insomnia the following night, thus contributing to further use of these medications. Although there are minimal data about the risks of prolonged benzodiazepine therapy, there are reports of increased risks of road traffic accidents among patients on these medications. Therefore, patients on prolonged therapy should be educated about these potential risks and told to avoid situations likely to increase them (e.g. mixing with alcohol, driving while sleepy).

Table 33 Commonly prescribed hypnotics

Medication	*Half life (h)*	*Dosage (mg)*
Benzodiazepines		
Midazolam	2–3	7.5–15
Triazolam	2–4	0.125–0.25
Brotizolam	4.5–6	0.125–0.5
Oxazepam	6–9	10–30
Temazepam	8–10	10–60
Lorazepam	8–12	0.5–20
Estazolam	14–18	0.5–20
Flunitrazepam	15–20	0.5–10
Clonazepam	20–25	0.5–2.0
Diazepam	20–50	5–10
Nitrazepam	25–50	2.5–10
Flurazepam	30–80	15–30
Sedatives (non-benzodiazepines)		
Zaleplon	1–1.5	5–20
Zolpidem	1.5–2.0	5–10
Zopiclone	4.5–5.5	3.75–7.5
Hypnotic antidepressants		
Trazodone	4–7	50–150
Amitriptyline	14–18	25–75
Doxepin	20–25	75–150

Non-benzodiazepine receptor agonists

Zaleplon (Sonata), zopiclone (Imovane) and zolpidem (Stilnox, Ambien) are three newly released medications, which work much like benzodiazepines. Although the chemical structure of the drugs is unrelated to that of classic benzodiazepines, they work at the same receptors as these medications. In clinical practice, these medications are essentially indistinguishable from true benzodiazepines. As zaleplon and zolpidem are quite short acting, we recommend their use as an alternative in clinical situations where a very short-acting benzodiazepine is indicated. Recent data suggest that the non-benzodiazepine receptor agonist may have fewer side effects and may be a better choice for intermittent use than benzodiazepines. Thus, they may be most appropriate for sleep initiation insomnia or as a hypnotic in the middle of the night in individuals with prolonged awakenings.

Sedating antidepressants

Sedating antidepressants are commonly used for the treatment of insomnia. At the present time in North America, the most commonly prescribed medication for inducing sleep is trazodone. Although there are minimal data to support its use, there has been excellent clinical experience with the use of this medication. There are some data suggesting a reduced risk of falls in elderly people who are given trazodone as opposed to tricyclic antidepressants and other SSRIs. There are minimal if any side effects with the use of this medication. However, there are two issues that should be addressed with the initiation of trazodone treatment: first, there is a rare complication of priapism (painful erection) that has been associated with trazodone in roughly 1 case per 5000 patients. Second, there has been an abstract presented in the cardiology community suggesting an increased risk of cardiac arrhythmias in patients receiving trazodone, as opposed to no medication and compared with SSRIs. These data were apparently based on statistical associations and have not yet been published in a peer-reviewed journal. We are currently awaiting publication of this manuscript before changing prescribing practices based on this study. However, patients should be informed of these data, as the lay press has spread this information and therefore patients may become alarmed upon hearing of these reports.

Insomnia: summary and patient approach

As discussed above, patients complaining of poor sleep (difficulties initiating and maintaining sleep) are classified as insomniacs. The initial approach to these patients is to consider the duration and the severity of the complaint (see Figure 16). Acute insomnia (<3 weeks) is generally

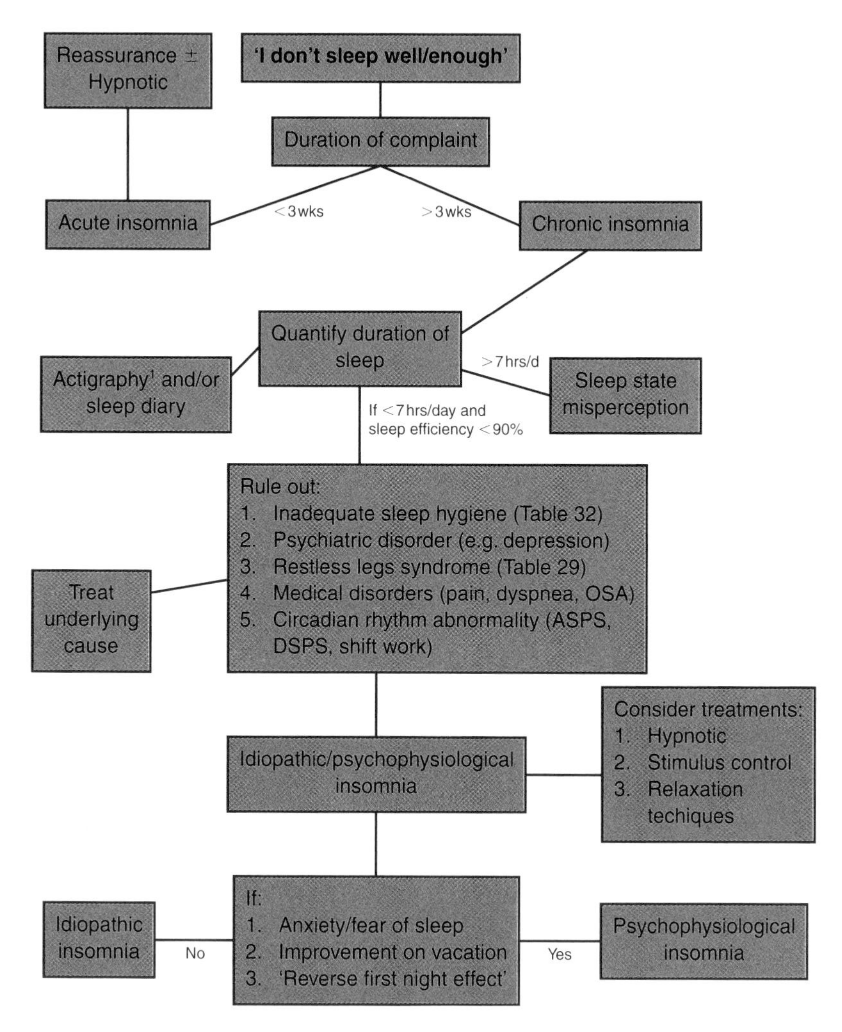

Figure 16 *Flowchart of the approach to the insomnia patient.*
[1]Actigraphy; a device to monitor sleep–wake behaviour by registering body movements.

self-limiting and can be treated with reassurance and/or with an hypnotic, particularly when the complaints started after a stressful life event. For the patient with chronic insomnia, quantification of sleep duration and sleep quality can be helpful using either actigraphy and/or sleep diaries. For patients who describe their duration and quality of sleep inaccurately, the diagnosis of sleep state misperception is made. In many of these patients, reassurance, supported by the objective sleep measures, may alleviate anxiety and reduce symptoms, and sometimes treatment of other causes of insomnia is required. For other patients, treatment of secondary aetiologies such as poor sleep hygiene, depression, sleep apnoea, nocturnal asthma, restless legs syndrome or other medical causes of insomnia, as well as circadian rhythm abnormalities, should be undertaken. Most of these diagnoses are made by the patient's history although in some specific cases objective tests are recommended, particularly if breathing disorders of sleep are suspected, and selectively in some cases of circadian rhythm disorders. The remainder of the patients, in whom no medical cause is found and sleep state misperception is ruled out, will have a diagnosis of either idiopathic or psychophysiological insomnia, which occasionally can be difficult to distinguish (see Table 28). Psychophysiological insomnia is generally associated with fear/anxiety regarding sleep and typically improves in foreign environments (e.g. on vacation or in the sleep laboratory). It is commonly presented in early adulthood. Idiopathic insomnia commonly lasts from early childhood, and is generally more difficult to treat. The treatment for this final group of insomnia patients (idiopathic/psychophysiological) is complex, and should generally be done by a sleep specialist. It usually consists of a combination of enforcing rules of sleep hygiene, cognitive behavioural therapy using techniques such as stimulus control, relaxation techniques, and hypnotic medications, separately or in combination (see text for details). When adequately performed, the reported success rate for this combined treatment ranges between 70–90%.

chapter 9

Parasomnias

The parasomnias are undesirable events that occur exclusively during the sleep period or that are exacerbated by sleep. Although some of the parasomnias may be quite frightening, most of them are benign, self-limited and only infrequently require treatment. Generally, the vast majority of the parasomnias are more common in children, although some of them tend to persist into adulthood or elderly life. There are several possible ways to classify the parasomnias. The most widely accepted classification is that suggested by the American Academy of Sleep Medicine, which is based on the sleep stage during which each of the parasomnias tends to occur (see Appendix).

The parasomnias in this book are discussed according to this classification.

Definition and classification

The parasomnias are a group of sleep disorders that consist of undesirable physical and behavioural phenomena which occur predominantly during sleep. Although these disorders intrude into or occur during sleep, they are not usually associated with a primary complaint of insomnia or excessive sleepiness. Most of the parasomnias can be diagnosed based on history alone, although in some cases the differential diagnosis is difficult and some further testing is required (usually polysomnography or PSG). The characteristics, diagnosis and approach to each of the specific parasomnias are classified according to the following four categories, based on the state in which they tend to occur:

1 The arousal disorders (which tend to occur in non-rapid eye movement [NREM] sleep)
2 The sleep–wake transition disorders
3 The parasomnias associated with REM sleep
4 Other parasomnias.

Disorders of arousal

Sleep terrors, sleep walking and confusional arousals are generally grouped as disorders of arousal. Sometimes sleep talking is included in this group as well, although it may occur during any sleep stage. These events generally occur out of deep NREM sleep (stages 3 and 4) and, thus, most often take place in the first third of the night when these sleep stages are most common. The patient is believed to be in a state between sleep and waking with some behavioural and EEG characteristics of each. Furthermore, inducing rapid arousals from slow wave sleep (SWS) can provoke these events. Actually any factor that deepens sleep or is associated with arousals may increase the occurrence of arousal disorders. These factors include recovery from sleep deprivation, sedative hypnotics, noisy sleep environment (causing arousals), obstructive sleep apnoea (OSA), etc. Some researchers believe that these three phenomena, i.e. sleep terrors, sleep walking and confusional awakenings, represent a single continuum ranging from confusional arousals with low motor and autonomic activation, on the one hand, to sleep walking characterized by intense motor activity and mild autonomic activation, on the other. According to this theory, night terrors fall between these two, with intense autonomic discharge and mild motor activation. Patients who experience one of these three phenomena are prone to demonstrate the others as well. Additional common features to these three phenomena include their increased prevalence in childhood and improvement with age, complete amnesia to the event in the morning after waking up from sleep, familial aggregation and frequently worsening after sleep deprivation. The common and differing features of the disorders of arousals are summarized in Tables 34 and 35.

During a confusional arousal event, a child may be disoriented and express odd behaviour. The child may be partially aware of the environment and thus may be confused and combine reality with imagination, e.g. the child may sit up in the bed and put a toy in his mouth thinking that it is a dummy/pacifier. Confusional arousals decrease with age, although they may still be seen in adults. As the events are benign, with almost no harmful consequences, in most cases no treatment is indicated. Avoidance of sleep deprivation and good sleep hygiene are recommended, as a rule of thumb, in all disorders of arousal.

Sleep walking

The events occurring during sleep walking are implied by the name. Actually, sleep walking, also known as somnambulism, can consist of very complex motor activity, of which walking is just one element. Sleep walkers have been reported to walk long distances, to conduct a variety of motor activities, and even to drive a car while sleep walking. In children, episodes of sleep walking are rarely violent. In adults, however, occasionally sleep walking may include violent gestures, which can endanger the patient or others. Such cases may turn into complicated legal issues in which sleep walking has been used as a possible explanation by the defence in homicide trials.

Table 34 Common features of the disorders of arousal

1	Tend to arise from slow wave sleep (stage 3–4)
2	A state between sleep and waking during the event, disorientation and confusion
3	Common in childhood
4	Decrease with increasing age
5	Cluster in families
6	Amnesia of the event
7	Can be precipitated by forced awakenings, worsens after sleep deprivation

Table 35 Characteristic features of the disorders of arousal

	Confusional arousals	*Sleep terrors*	*Sleep walking*
Behaviour	Inappropriate, weird	Screaming, crying, intense fear	Walking, talking
Prevalence	Very common under 5 years of age, may persist into adulthood	3–4% in children, less than 1% in adults	Peak age 4–8 years, when prevalence is 20% In adults 3–4%
Male : female ratio	1 : 1	Males > females	1 : 1
Motor activity	Low	Rarely complex	Complex
Autonomic activity	Low	Intense	Mild
Complications	Rare (aggressiveness)	Occasional (escape)	Possible (violence)
Treatment	Avoid precipitating factors, reassurance	Avoid precipitating factors, safety, benzodiazepines	Avoid precipitating factors, safety, benzodiazepines

Sleep walking is very common during childhood. The reported prevalence varies according to the definition used (i.e. the frequency of events), and ranges between 15 and 30% in children, and between 1 and 4% in adults. Most adults who sleep walk also had episodes of sleep walking during childhood, although not all. The familial history is very important, because the prevalence in children increases to 45% if one parent was affected, and to 60% if both. Its possible genetic origin is also supported by the fact that the concordance rate in monozygotic twins is 55% compared with 35% in dizygotic twins. As with all disorders of arousal, the sleep walking events tend to occur in the first third of the night (when most of the SWS occurs). This is more true in children, because in adults recent studies reported the occurrence of sleep-walking episodes in sleep stage 2 throughout the night. In the morning, patients typically have complete amnesia for the event. During the event, the eyes are usually open, but the expression is dull or glassy. Events may last from several minutes to an hour.

Somnambulism may be precipitated by a variety of conditions such as sleep deprivation, fever, stress, medications (phenothiazines, chloral hydrate, lithium) and other disorders that result in arousals (OSA, distended bladder, loud noise). Previous studies reported that persistence of sleep walking into adulthood is a marker of psychopathology. However, several recent studies have questioned this assertion and reported no clear association between psychopathology and somnambulism. It is postulated that in some cases the re-experiencing of sleep walking after several years of remission may result from chronic partial sleep deprivation which is common in young adults in developed countries.

Simple sleep walking usually does not require specific treatment other than safety precautions (i.e. lock doors and windows, remove hazardous objects, etc.) and avoidance of precipitating factors. In some cases additional treatment may be considered. Such circumstances may include a very high frequency of events, suspected psychosocial complications (e.g. if a child avoids 'sleep-overs' with friends), or when events are violent and potentially injurious. In these cases a low-dose benzodiazepine is the drug of choice (clonazepam, temazepam, triazolam, brotizolam, lorazepam, diazepam), although tricyclic antidepressants and trazodone may be beneficial as well. In some cases behavioural therapy such as hypnosis can be successful.

Diagnosis is usually easily established by history only. In some cases of non-typical history, very complex stereotypical automatism or unusual behaviours, seizures (especially frontal or temporal lobe epilepsy or partial complex seizures) should be suspected. In these cases a PSG with video recording is indicated. Even without experiencing an event in the laboratory, some PSG findings are suggestive of sleep walking. These include increased SWS, hypersynchronized EEG δ activity, and frequent stage shifts from SWS to shallow sleep or arousals. Electrical discharges in the EEG are obviously suggestive of some sort of epilepsy. Other differential diagnoses include other movement disorders of sleep such as REM behavioural disorder (see below), periodic limb movement disorder (PLMD), paroxysmal nocturnal dystonia (very similar to frontal lobe epilepsy) or dissociative states.

Lady Macbeth sleep walking

Gentlewoman: Since his Majesty went into the field, I have seen her rise from her bed, throw her night-gown upon her, unlock her closet, take forth paper, fold it, write upon't, read it, afterwards seal it, and again return to bed; yet all this while in a most fast sleep.

Doctor: A great perturbation in nature, to receive at once the benefit of sleep and do the effects of watching! In this slumb'ry agitation, besides her walking and other actual performances, what, at any time, have you heard her say?

Gentlewoman: That, sir, which I will not report after her.

Doctor: You may to me, and 'tis most meet you should.

Gentlewoman: Neither to you nor any one, having no witness to confirm my speech.

(*Enter Lady Macbeth with a taper*)

Lo you, here she comes! This is her very guise, and upon my life, fast asleep. Observe her, stand close.

Doctor: How came she by that light?

> Gentlewoman: Why it stood by her. She has light by her continually, 'tis her command.
> Doctor: You see her eyes are open.
> Gentlewoman: Ay, but their sense are shut.
> Doctor: What is it she does now? Look how she rubs her hands.
> Gentlewoman: It is an accustom'd action with her, to seem thus washing her hands. I have known her continue in this a quarter of an hour . . .
> Doctor: This disease is beyond my practice: yet I have known those which have walk'd in their sleep who have died holily in their beds.
>
> William Shakespeare, *Macbeth*.

Sleep terrors

Sleep terrors are characterized by the sudden arousal from sleep with a heart-breaking scream and intense fear manifested by heightened sympathetic activation (tachycardia, diaphoresis, flushing of the skin, mydriasis and hyperpnoea). Although during the recording of an event the muscular electromyograph (EMG) increases as well, true motor activity is usually absent. However, occasionally, attempts to 'escape' may be associated with movements, potentially injurious. The typical age is 4–12 (peak at 5–7), with an approximate prevalence of 3–4% in this age group, which declines to less than 1% in adults. During an event, the child is unresponsive and confused as in other disorders of arousal. Once fully alert, the child generally has amnesia about the sleep event, and does not have a recollection of a dream. This is one of the classic differences between sleep terrors and nightmares (Table 36). The distinction between them may be important for prognostic and further evaluation purposes, i.e. in cases of recurrent nightmares a psychological evaluation may be indicated to rule out stress, trauma (abuse) or personality disorders, whereas in sleep terrors sometimes EEG recording is required to rule out temporal or frontal lobe epilepsy. As with other disorders of arousal, therapy is directed towards avoidance of precipitating factors

Table 36 Different characteristics of sleep terrors and nightmares

Sleep terrors	*Nightmares*
From SWS (first third of the night)	From REM sleep (last third of the night)
Heart-breaking cry, screams	Scary awakening
Disoriented, confused	Awakens from the event, then fully alert
Common vocalization	Rare vocalization
Extreme sympathetic discharge	Mild–moderate sympathetic activation
Amnesia of the event	Awareness of the event
No recollection of dream	Dream recall (scary vivid dream)
Males (M) > females (F)	In children M = F, in adults F > M
Age 4–12 (peak at 5–7)	Any age (frequent at age 3–6)
3–4% in children, <1% in adults	10–20% in children, up to 5% in adults
Familial history present	Familial history absent
Potentially injurious and violent	Rarely injurious or violent
Predisposing: fever, sleep deprivation	Stress, traumatic events, personality disorders
Treatment: safety, avoid predisposing factors, benzodiazepines	None, psycho/behavioural therapy

SWS, slow wave sleep.

and establishment of environmental precautions (locking doors, sleeping at a lower level, etc.). Only rarely are low-dose benzodiazepines indicated.

Sleep–wake transition disorders

Sleep starts and sleep talking

The sleep–wake transition disorders are a group of events that may occur during the wake-to-sleep transition, sleep-to-wake transition or rarely also during transitions from one sleep stage to another. Some of them are so obvious, common and benign that they are considered a normal phenomenon and not a disorder. An example of this is the *sleep starts*, which consist of muscle jerks or abrupt movement of the limbs or head, associated with the sensation of falling, at sleep onset. One potential explanation for this is a rapid loss of muscle tone, just before the wake-to-sleep transition, which elicits a reflex response of sharp firing of muscles to restore the tone. This phenomenon may occur at any age, and actually happens occasionally in most individuals.

Likewise, *sleep talking* (somniloquy) is also very common and may be considered as physiological rather than pathological. The clinical range is wide, from just odd sounds, through chains of unrelated words, to a long 'speech'. Although considered a sleep–wake transition disorder, it can occur during continuous sleep and is very common in association with the disorders of arousal (which are also conditions with partial wakefulness, see above).

Both sleep starts and sleep talking need no treatment, unless they are very frequent, to the point where they cause sleep disturbances to the bed partner. Sometimes they can result in embarrassment or increased anxiety, in which case a therapeutic trial of sleep restriction may be considered. Sleep restriction may shorten the period of transition from wake to sleep, and by increasing the homoeostatic sleep drive can improve all disorders of sleep–wake transition.

Rhythmic movement disorder

There is no doubt that the most impressive wake-to-sleep transition disorder is the rhythmic movement disorder (RMD). Rhythmic, stereotypical movements of the head, trunk and extremities, generally on falling asleep, manifest this parasomnia. It is well described in otherwise healthy children, with an overall prevalence of up to 5% of children, with a boy : girl ratio of 4 : 1. These movements are thought to help the child with sleep onset, in a similar way to relaxation. The natural history of this phenomenon is to decrease in frequency and intensity, but it is not rare to persist into adulthood.

The term 'rhythmic movement disorders' was initially introduced for these repetitive movements in sleep, which may appear as head banging (jactatio capitis), body rocking or leg rolling. However, some rare forms of RMD have been reported, e.g. a case of a healthy 2-year-old girl with repeated nocturnal tongue biting. The distinction from nocturnal seizures in such cases may be crucial to avoid overtreatment with anti-epileptic agents.

This disorder is considered benign, albeit sometimes rather dramatic and frightening. Severe injuries have been reported, including fractures, subdural effusions and eye injuries, depending on the characteristic movement. It may increase with stress or as a result of lack of stimulation. For this reason, it is seen more frequently in neglected children. The prevalence is also higher among children with pervasive developmental disorder (autism) or psychomotor retardation. Treatment, again, should include sleep hygiene instructions and attempts to restrict sleep. Obviously sleep environment should be suitably altered (i.e. upholster the bed and its banister).

Nocturnal leg cramps

Finally, nocturnal leg cramps are also considered to be a sleep–wake transition disorder. This phenomenon describes the awakenings from sleep with sensation of pain in the calves or feet. Muscle tension may also occur. It occurs mainly in adults, and more frequently in women. Over the years, several predisposing factors have been recognized, including vigorous exercise, pregnancy and contraceptive use. In addition, it occurs more commonly in patients with neuromuscular diseases, chronic arthritis, Parkinson's disease or diabetes mellitus. Electrolyte imbalances such as hypocalcaemia may also predispose an individual to experience nocturnal leg cramps. As with all sleep–wake transition disorders diagnosis is usually made by the history alone. PSG is not required but, if performed, EEG is normal and the EMG may show non-periodic bursts (as opposed to PLMs). Usually the events need no treatment unless they are very frequent or lead to unbearable pain or anxiety. In such cases, muscle relaxants may be used (e.g. baclofen). Additional therapy such as a hot bath, massage or relaxation treatment may also be helpful. If it results in insomnia, clonazepam may be considered.

Parasomnias associated with REM sleep

As discussed before, unique features such as muscle atonia, rapid eye movements, EEG activation, dreams and penile erection in males characterize REM sleep. Each one of these characteristics, when occurring at undesired times, or abnormally, can result in parasomnia. These are grouped together as REM-related parasomnias. The common pathophysiological process in all these parasomnias is that they either occur exclusively during REM sleep or have REM sleep features and occur at various times.

Nightmares

Nightmares are frightening dreams that usually awaken the individual from REM sleep, which can be recalled after the awakening. Similar to sleep terrors it can also be manifested as a sudden nocturnal event associated with a cry, sensation of fear, some autonomic activation and abnormal movements. However, classically it differs from sleep terrors in many ways (see Table 36). When awakened from a nightmare, the individual is usually fully alert and oriented, and can recall a bad/scary dream. Movements during an event are quite rare because of the REM-related skeletal muscle atonia. Nightmares are generally not associated with violent outbursts, no displacement from the bed occurs and injuries are uncommon. Return to sleep is delayed, and the individual is usually alert and may desire to converse.

Although everyone may have occasional bad dreams, the dreams defined as nightmares are characterized by being associated with an immediate threat to the individual's security, self-esteem or survival. The aetiology of nightmares is not very well understood. Although sporadic nightmares may be normal responses to stress, chronic nightmares can be troublesome and represent an underlying disorder. Frequent nightmares may be associated with abnormal psychological tests and psychiatric disorders (as opposed to sleep terrors which only rarely reflect underlying pathology). Recurrent nightmares should raise the suspicion of post-traumatic stress disorder (PTSD). The onset of nightmares in an adult is often associated with medication, illness or severely stressful events. Sedatives/hypnotics, β blockers, amphetamines and dopamine agonists have been reported to result in nightmares.

The prevalence differs among researchers according to the definition used. Recurrent disturbing nightmares are reported to occur in 10–20% of children, and up to 5% of adults. The peak age in children is between ages 3 and 6 years, without any sex bias or clear familial pattern. In adults, however, nightmares are substantially more common in women than men.

The diagnosis is usually made by history alone (see Table 36). In unclear or atypical cases PSG may be indicated, which may reveal an abrupt arousal or repeated arousals from REM sleep, with mild–moderate sympathetic activation. When no event occurs during the night of PSG, suggestive features may include short REM onset, increased portion of REM sleep out of total sleep time and particularly increased REM density (increased number of eye movements per minute of REM sleep). Unlike REM behavioural disorder (see below), the submental EMG in nightmares shows decreased activity (atonia) and, unlike seizures, the EEG is normal.

When considering treatment for nightmares several factors have to be considered. First, many cases need no treatment (depending on the intensity, frequency and consequences of events). Second, if there is an underlying disorder (such as PTSD or psychosis), treatment should be directed at the primary disorder and not the result. However, recent studies in crime victims who suffered from nightmares showed that behavioural treatment aimed at altering the nightmare content towards more positive emotional imageries significantly improved patients' sleep. If nightmares are diagnosed without an underlying disorder, and a decision is made to apply treatment, psychotherapy is the preferred approach. Only rarely may medications such as antipsychotics or antidepressants be considered.

Sleep paralysis

Although sleep paralysis may occur during the transition from wakefulness to sleep or from sleep to wakefulness, it is considered to be a REM-related parasomnia for two reasons. First, it tends to occur during awakenings from REM sleep. Second, its pathophysiology probably involves the REM-related atonia. As with the normal physiology during REM sleep, sleep paralysis is characterized by atonia of skeletal muscles, with areflexia. Individuals are unable to move their limbs, head and trunk, although respiration and eye movements remain normal. It occurs frequently after arousal from REM sleep, and it is postulated that it is caused by cortical awakening before the termination of REM-related atonia. A sleep paralysis episode may last seconds to minutes and terminates either spontaneously or through an external stimulus such as a sound or a touch. Patients usually describe these episodes as frightening or even terrifying because they are fully awake and conscious, yet unable to move. It can be either an isolated problem or a part of the narcolepsy syndrome (see Chapter 6). The isolated form may be familial. Many people experience at least one episode in a lifetime (about 30–50% of normal individuals). However, chronic recurrent episodes that are not associated with narcolepsy are relatively uncommon (a prevalence of less than 1%). Sleep paralysis episodes occur more frequently after sleep deprivation and sleep–wake schedule problems (shift work, jet lag, delayed sleep phase syndrome).

Several other conditions should be considered in the differential diagnosis, such as cataplexy, seizure, psychotic state and periodic paralysis. Unlike cataplexy, it is not provoked by emotions, and does not occur out of a fully awake state. Seizures should also be considered in the differential diagnosis. In addition to the abnormal movements seen during seizure activity and the abnormal EEG, the termination of a sleep paralysis is usually abrupt with a quick transition to full wakefulness, whereas in seizures a post-ictal sleepiness is common. A psychotic state is usually easy to distinguish from sleep paralysis from the history and other indications of the psychiatric profile of the patient. Periodic paralysis caused by a potassium imbalance may be difficult to distinguish from sleep paralysis. This problem may result from either hypokalaemia or hyperkalaemia, usually has a familial pattern, and is seen primarily in children and adolescents. It can be provoked by vigorous exercise and by glucose administration (the hypokalaemic form). It also often occurs at the transition from sleep to wakefulness, so examination of serum potassium level may be indicated. Hypokalaemic or hyperkalaemic periodic paralysis may be treated with acetazolamide. Potassium chloride should be given during hypokalaemic episodes.

Sleep paralysis itself does not usually require any particular treatment (i.e. unless it is associated with narcolepsy). Avoiding predisposing factors such as sleep deprivation and treating circadian rhythm abnormalities may be of benefit. In rare cases of frequent prolonged frightening episodes, antidepressants may be given.

REM sleep behavioural disorder

REM sleep behavioural disorder (RBD) is characterized by a disinhibition of the normal muscle atonia associated with REM sleep. As a result, dreams can be 'acted out', and movements are quite often violent and injurious to self or the bed partner. Patients can often recall dreams after the event. The exact prevalence of this condition is unclear, but recent studies suggest that it might not be an uncommon condition. Elderly people are affected more often and there is a male preponderance. RBD is thought to result from dysfunction of the brain-stem mechanisms responsible for suppression of motor tone during REM sleep. Although transient RBD can be seen after taking certain drugs or during drug withdrawal, the chronic type is usually idiopathic or associated with an underlying degenerative neurological condition. Diseases associated with RBD include Parkinson's disease (and may be the initial manifestation), chronic alcohol abuse, dementia and the use of REM-suppressing medications.

PSG recording typically shows elevated tonic and phasic EMG tone during REM sleep. Differential diagnosis includes other abnormal movements during sleep. These may result from seizures, PLMs, sleep walking/night terrors, nightmares (PTSD) and nocturnal panic attacks. OSA should also be considered in the differential diagnosis because apnoeas during REM sleep may result in awakenings with increased EMG and limb movements. However, OSA is usually easily distinguished from RBD by both history and PSG. REM behavioural disorder, in contrast to the disorders of arousal (sleep walking and sleep terrors), evolves out of REM sleep and, thus, tends to occur in the final third of the night when REM sleep is most common.

Also, in RBD dream recall is very common unlike the disorders of arousal. Although the typical age of the disorders of arousals is childhood, the typical age of RBD onset is 50–60 years. Nightmares may be very difficult to distinguish from RBD. Both arise from REM sleep and may be associated with terrifying dreams and violent movements. However, complex movements are uncommon in nightmares. In addition, the typical PSG finding in RBD is increased EMG during REM sleep, whereas in nightmares the EMG is usually low and only the REM density increases (frequent eye movements). Finally, seizures may also be considered in the differential diagnosis, although the movements are typically stereotypical and the EEG shows no abnormal electrical discharges. As about one-third of cases of RBD arise from an underlying neurological abnormality (such as Parkinson's disease, multiple sclerosis, subarachnoid haemorrhage, dementia, neoplasm or cerebrovascular disease), extensive evaluation, including a thorough neurological examination, magnetic resonance imaging (MRI) and full clinical EEG are recommended. Careful longitudinal follow-up is also recommended because RBD can precede the onset of other neurological diseases.

Therapy is usually indicated given the potential for injury. Clonazepam has been the most extensively used agent and is effective in most cases at a dose of 0.5–2.0 mg. Other, shorter-acting benzodiazepines may be of value if daytime sedation is a problem. Environmental precautions are also required.

Impaired/painful nocturnal erections

It has been well known, for many years, that episodic, periodic, nocturnal erections occur during sleep in every male at every age. In fact, this was known well before REM sleep was discovered. Only in the late 1960s was the linkage between nocturnal erections and REM sleep discovered. However, it should be mentioned that it is not clear whether the erections during REM sleep are caused by underlying REM-related mechanisms, or are independently generated and just synchronized with the REM episodes, e.g. periodic erections have been reported to persist in a patient with almost no REM sleep (as a result of pontine injury). Penile erection is primarily a parasympathetic process, involving efferent neural flow from the sacral plexus S2, S3, S4, resulting in arterial vasodilatation of the penile artery. Thus penile erection is a relative exception in light of otherwise sympathetic dominance during REM sleep.

The functional significance of nocturnal erections is unknown, although, along with the other components of the 'stimulation' theory of REM sleep, it has been suggested that the brain periodically activates this complex system during REM sleep, in order to be able to use it while awake (i.e. 'use it or lose it concept'). Regardless of its purpose, measuring penile erections during sleep has a clinical significance, because impotence largely consists of about 50% psychological causes and 50% somatic ones. Absence of REM-related erections supports an organic aetiology (secondary to injury, diabetes, hypertension, medications, or other vascular or neural problems), whereas intact REM-related erections yield psychological aetiology of impotence. It should be mentioned that drawing conclusions from measuring penile tumescence or rigidity alone without any reference to sleep is not sufficient, because erections are seen usually only in REM periods that are longer than 10 minutes and are not fragmented. Therefore, penile tumescence or rigidity measurements should be performed simultaneously with a full PSG to detect sleep pattern and REM sleep periods, and to rule out sleep fragmentation. If not performed, absence of nocturnal erections secondary to sleep fragmentation may be misdiagnosed as an organic cause for impotence, which may lead to the wrong treatment.

Thus, although 'impaired sleep-related penile erections' is listed as a sleep disorder from the parasomnia group, it is a physiological somatic disorder indicating organic impotence, and has no direct effect on sleep as such. On the other hand, 'sleep-related painful erections' may certainly lead to a sleep disorder, as a result of REM fragmentation. In this rare disorder, men occasionally wake up from REM sleep with painful erections, although their erections during wakefulness are painless. If frequent and common, anatomical abnormalities of the penis should be ruled out (e.g. Peyronie's disease). As this is a very rare disorder, little is known about its treatment. Surprisingly, REM-suppressor medications such as antidepressants have been reported to be ineffective. The antipsychotic dibenzodiazepine, clozapine, as well as the β blocker, propranolol, have been reported to result in a favourable response.

Other parasomnias

This category of parasomnias consists of all parasomnias that did not fit into one of the above categories. Although several parasomnias are listed there, only bruxism and enuresis are discussed here. Nocturnal paroxysmal dystonia is briefly mentioned under the differential diagnosis of sleep-walking, and primary snoring is actually a very mild form of sleep-disordered breathing (see Chapters 5 and 6). Infant sleep apnoea and congenital central hypoventilation syndrome are neonatal problems and not discussed in this book.

Bruxism

Sleep bruxism is a stereotypical movement disorder characterized by grinding or clenching of the teeth during sleep. The disorder may often occur in otherwise healthy normal individuals, and may come to clinical attention because of a complaint from a bed partner. In fact, most of the population will at some time during their lifetime experience bruxism. It becomes pathological when it is associated with other phenomena, such as insomnia caused by sleep fragmentation, dental damage, jaw pain, masseter muscle hypertrophy or temporomandibular joint (TMJ) problems. The exact prevalence is hard to determine because many people are unaware of having the disorder. In about 5% of the population, it may represent a clinical problem, although it may occur in up to 6–12% of adults as a chronic disorder. Bruxism seems to appear more frequently in the younger population and to decline with increasing age.

The aetiology and pathophysiology of the disorder are unknown. However, some predisposing factors are recognized, including tooth interference in dental occlusion, stress, anxiety and possibly neurological disorders (mainly those involving the dopaminergic system). When bruxism produces sufficient noise to disturb the bed partner or when any of the consequences mentioned above are noted, a formal diagnosis and treatment are recommended. PSG typically shows repeated, phasic increases in jaw muscles (submental EMG), best seen over the masseters, but frequently noted also in the EEG channels. The general sleep pattern is usually normal. The bruxing episodes may occur at any sleep stage, although they are more likely to occur in light sleep, REM sleep and sleep–wake transitions. For this reason, rhythmic movement of sleep should also be considered in the differential diagnosis.

At this time, there is no curative treatment that results in abolishing oromotor activity. Treatment should focus on relieving symptoms and preventing permanent sequelae. Three types of management strategies have been used: dental, pharmacological and psychobehavioural. Evaluation by a dentist is recommended. Adjustment of tooth bite or occlusion, or using an intraoral appliance (either a soft mouth-guard or a hard plastic bite splint), may protect the teeth, alleviate pain, minimize TMJ dysfunction and potentially reduce oromotor activity. Muscle relaxants and benzodiazepines have been reported to improve sleep bruxism, although the scientific data for this are lacking. Benzodiazepines may certainly improve sleep continuity but dependence and daytime drowsiness may develop.

Psychobehavioural treatment, such as biofeedback, aversive conditioning and other relaxation techniques (e.g. hypnosis), may reduce stress and anxiety and provide some relief. Finally, improving sleep hygiene and avoiding coffee or other stimulant substances in the afternoon should also be recommended.

Enuresis

Nocturnal enuresis or 'bed-wetting' is a common problem in children, with a prevalence of approximately 7–15% of boys at 5 years of age, 3–5% at age 10 and about 1% of men. In women the disorder is less common, and is estimated to be 3–5% at age 5, about 2% at age 10 and uncommon in adult women. The term 'nocturnal enuresis' refers to patients who control urination well during wakefulness, but have isolated nocturnal enuresis. It should be distinguished from nocturia, which refers to the need to urinate during the night, but with the patient waking up to urinate in the bathroom rather than bed-wetting.

Common causes of nocturia include benign prostatic hyperplasia, diuretic therapy and glucosuria. Previously it was common to differentiate between primary (having never been continent) and secondary enuresis (developing after at least a 6-month period of continence). However, more recent practice shows that both can arise from either organic or functional causes, and the distinction between primary and secondary enuresis has a low (if any) clinical value. Nevertheless, in children most cases are primary (75%), and often result from inadequate or inappropriate toilet training. Secondary enuresis often results from a stressful event such as the birth of a sibling. Although most nocturnal enuresis cases are functional, many organic causes of nocturnal enuresis have been documented. These include a variety of anatomical and functional genitourinary abnormalities, chronic pelvic/urinary infection, chronic constipation, diseases associated with polyuria (diabetes mellitus or insipidus), lack of nocturnal rise of antidiuretic hormone, seizure activity, and very deep sleep with blunted arousal response. This final cause is relatively common in chronic sleep deprivation conditions such as in sleep apnoea syndrome. Indeed, nocturnal enuresis is significantly more common in children with OSA, although alternative mechanisms such as sympathetic activation have been proposed. Finally, genetics also probably plays a role, because nocturnal enuresis tends to be familial. Nocturnal enuresis may occur at any time during the night, in any sleep stage.

Although the vast majority of cases of nocturnal enuresis are functional, diagnostic evaluation can exclude organic causes. Usually careful history taking is very helpful and can help to rule out the possibility of previous urinary tract infections, OSA or other sleep disorders, and epilepsy. Physical examination should be focused on detection of neurological abnormalities. Urinalysis, urine culture and voiding function (including residual volume after voiding and urinary flow measurements) are occasionally indicated. However, again, most cases are idiopathic with no other abnormality detected.

The therapeutic approach to the child with nocturnal enuresis should begin with appropriate education and sleep hygiene regulations. There are several steps that should be taken:

1. Treat primary cause if found (somatic or emotional)
2. Avoid drinking after dinner
3. Always void before retiring to bed
4. Educate the child about the consequences of the bed-wetting; the child should launder his or her soiled bed sheets and clothes (not as a punishment)
5. Generally, rewarding is preferable to punishing. Children should be rewarded for dry nights. Punishment or humiliation of the child should be avoided.

When these steps fail, other treatments should be considered. First, it should be kept in mind that the spontaneous cure rate in children is approximately 15% per year. Treatment options include pharmacological therapy or behavioural conditioning. The commonly used medications are tricyclic antidepressants (mostly imipramine, working primarily on its anticholinergic effects), and desmopressin, an analogue of antidiuretic hormone (vasopressin, working by increasing reabsorption of water in the kidney and inhibiting urine production during the night). Although both of these medications are helpful when administered, enuresis frequently recurs when the drugs are stopped, and often even close to the spontaneous cure rate (Table 37). Therefore, they are recommended mainly as an acute treatment, e.g. when a child goes to a sleep-over with friends (mainly desmopressin via nasal spray).

Table 37 Long-term treatment outcome of children with nocturnal enuresis

	Outcome	
	At the end of 1 year of treatment (%)	*After cessation of treatment (%)*
No treatment	15	15
Imipramine (25 mg)	50	30
Desmospray (20 μg)	90	20
Wet alarm	80	70

Conditioning therapy, on the other hand, is directed at teaching the child to deal with the enuresis on a long-term basis. It consists of an alarm system attached to a pad, which awakens the child when the first drops of urine are detected. Although this system takes several weeks to work, it can be highly successful (>70%) and provides the best long-term control of enuresis. Following this treatment, children often wake up to void instead of bed-wetting, and they occasionally report that they 'heard' the bell ringing even though the alarm system is no longer attached.

The numbers in Table 37 represent the approximate percentage of children in each group who become continent during treatment and remain so after treatment termination.

Appendix

International classification of sleep disorders

This classification groups the primary sleep disorders under two subgroups: the dyssomnias, which include those disorders that produce a complaint of insomnia or excessive sleepiness, and the parasomnias, which include those disorders that intrude into or occur during sleep but do not produce a primary complaint of insomnia or excessive sleepiness. The dyssomnias are further subdivided, in part along pathophysiological lines, into the intrinsic (induced primarily by factors within the body), extrinsic (induced primarily by factors outside the body) and circadian rhythm sleep disorders. The primary sleep disorders (dyssomnias and parasomnias) are separated from the medical/psychiatric sleep disorder section to remain compatible with the medical ICD (*International Classification of Diseases*). Finally, there is a fourth section of the ICSD which includes sleep disorders that could not be sufficiently classified into one of the other categories, usually as a result of inadequate or insufficient information available to substantiate the unequivocal existence of the disorder.

The following is a short list of some important diagnoses with their ICSD code:

Dyssomnias

A. Intrinsic sleep disorders

Psychophysiological insomnia	307.42-0
Sleep state misperception	307.49-1
Idiopathic insomnia	780.52-7

Narcolepsy	347
Recurrent hypersomnia	780.54-2
Idiopathic hypersomnia	780.54-7
Post-traumatic hypersomnia	780.54-8
Obstructive sleep apnoea syndrome	780.53-0
Central sleep apnoea syndrome	780.51-0
Central alveolar hypoventilation syndrome	780.51-1
Periodic limb movement disorder	780.52-4
Restless legs syndrome	780.52-5
B. Extrinsic sleep disorders	
Inadequate sleep hygiene	307.41-1
Environmental sleep disorder	780.52-6
Adjustment sleep disorder	307.41-0
Insufficient sleep syndrome	307.49-4
Limit-setting sleep disorder	307.42-4
Sleep-onset associated disorder	307.42-5
Food allergy insomnia	780.52-2
Nocturnal eating (drinking) syndrome	780.52-8
C. Circadian sleep disorders	
Shift work sleep disorder	307.45-1
Irregular sleep–wake pattern	307.45-3
Delayed sleep phase syndrome	780.55-0
Advanced sleep phase syndrome	780.55-1
Non-24-hour sleep–wake disorder	780.55-2

Parasomnias

A. Arousal disorders	
Confusional arousals	307.46-2
Sleep-walking	307.46-0
Sleep terrors	307.46-1
B. Sleep–wake transition disorders	
Rhythmic movement disorder	307.3
Sleep starts	307.47-2
Nocturnal leg cramps	729.82

C. Parasomnias usually associated with REM sleep	
Nightmares	307.47-0
Sleep paralysis	780.56-2
Impaired sleep-related penile erections	780.56-3
REM-sleep behavioural disorder	780.59-0
D. Other parasomnias	
Sleep bruxism	306.8
Sleep enuresis	780.56-0
Nocturnal paroxysmal dystonia	780.59-1
Primary snoring	780.53-1
Infant sleep apnoea	770.80
Congenital central hypoventilation syndrome	770.81

Sleep disorders associated with medical/psychiatric disorders

A. Associated with mental disorder	290-319
Psychoses	292-299
Mood disorders	296-301
Anxiety disorders	300
Panic disorders	300
Alcoholism	303
B. Associated with neurological disorders	320-389
Cerebral degenerative disorders	330-337
Dementia	331
Parkinsonism	332-333
Fatal familial insomnia	337.9
Sleep-related epilepsy	345
Electrical status epilepticus of sleep	345.8
Sleep-related headaches	346
C. Associated with other medical disorders	
Sleeping sickness	086
Nocturnal cardiac ischaemia	411-414
Chronic obstructive pulmonary disease	490-494
Sleep-related asthma	493
Sleep-related gastro-oesophageal reflux	530.1

Peptic ulcer disease	531-534
Fibrositis syndrome	729.1
Proposed sleep disorders	
Short sleeper	307.49-0
Long sleeper	307.49-2
Sleep-related laryngospasm	780.59-4
Sleep choking syndrome	307.42-1

References

Aserinsky E, Kleitman N. Regularly occurring periods of eye motility, and concomitant phenomena, during sleep. *Science* 1953; 118:273–4.

Benington JH, Heller HC. Implications of sleep deprivation experiments for our understanding of sleep homeostasis. *Sleep* 1999; 22(8):1033–43.

Berger H. Ueber das elektroenkephalogramm des Menschen. *J Psychol Neurol* 1930; 40:160–79.

Bremer F. Cerveau isole et physiologie du sommeil. *C R Soc Biol* 1935; 118:1235–41.

Caton R. Sleep of an obese poulterer. *Clin Soc Trans* 1889; 22:133–7.

Daniels L. Narcolepsy. *Medicine* 1934; 1–122.

Hedner J. Daytime waking autonomic function and vascular control in OSA. *J Sleep Res* 1995; 4:171–5.

Horner RL. Autonomic consequences of arousal from sleep: mechanisms and implications. *Sleep* 1996; 19:S193–5.

Jouvet M, Mounier D. Effects des lesions de la formation reticulaire pontique sur le sommeil du chat. *C R Soc Biol* 1960; 154:2301–5.

Legendre R, Pieron H. Le probleme des facteurs du sommeil. *C R Soc Biol* 1910; 68:1077–9.

Moruzzi G, Magoun H. Brain stem reticular formation and activation of the EEG. *Electroencephalog Clin Neurophysiol* 1949; 1:455–73.

Parmeggiani PL. Brain cooling across wake–sleep behavioural states in homeothermic species: an analysis of the underlying physiological mechanisms. *Rev Neurosci* 1995; 6:353–63.

Von Economo C. *Encephalitis Lethargica: Its Sequelae and Treatment.* Oxford University Press, London, 1931.

Zamboni G, Perez E, Amici R, Jones CA, Parmeggiani PL. Control of REM sleep: an aspect of the regulation of physiological homeostasis. *Arch Ital Biol* 1999; 137:249–62.

Further reading

Sleep, general

Bonnet MH, Arand DL. We are chronically sleep deprived. *Sleep* 1995; 18:908–11.

Brzezinski A. Melatonin in humans. *N Engl J Med* 1997; 336:186–95.

Dement WC, Vaughan C. *The Promise of Sleep : A Pioneer in Sleep Medicine Explores the Vital Connection Between Health, Happiness, and a Good Night's Sleep.* Delacorte, NY, 1999.

Dinges DF, Douglas SD, Hamarman S, Zaugg L, Kapoor S. Sleep deprivation and human immune function. *Adv Neuroimmunol* 1995; 5:97–110.

Ferrera M, De Gennaro L. How much sleep do we need? *Sleep Med Rev* 2001; 5: 155–179.

Jouvet M. *The Paradox of Sleep.* MIT Press, Boston, 2001.

Lavie P. *The Enchanted World of Sleep*. Yale University Press, New Haven, London, 1996.
Lin JS. Brain structures and mechanisms involved in the control of cortical activation and wakefulness, with emphasis on the posterior hypothalamus and histaminergic neurons. *Sleep Med Rev* 2001; 4:471–503.
Lugaresi E, Parmeggiani PL. *Somatic and Autonomic Regulation in Sleep: Physiological and Clinical Aspects*. Springer Verlag, Berlin, Heidelberg, 1997.
McGinty D, Szymusiak R. Brain structures and mechanisms involved in the generation of NREM sleep: focus on the preoptic hypothalamus. *Sleep Med Rev* 2001; 5:323–42.
Moore B. Circadian rhythms: basic neurobiology and clinical applications. *Annu Rev Med* 1997, 48:253–66.
Ogilvie RD. The process of falling asleep. *Sleep Med Rev* 2001; 5:247–70.
Orr WC. Gastrointestinal functioning during sleep: a new horizon in sleep medicine. *Sleep Med Rev* 2001; 5:91–101.
Reinoso-Suárez F, de Andrés I, Rodrigo-Angulo ML, Garzón M. Brain structures and mechanisms involved in the generation of REM sleep. *Sleep Med Rev* 2001; 5:63–77.
Shochat T, Haimov I, Lavie P. Melatonin – the key to the gate of sleep. *Ann Med* 1998; 30:109–14.
White DP. Complex home monitoring. *Sleep* 1996; 19:S248–50.

Sleep disorders, general

Chokroverty S. Diagnosis and treatment of sleep disorders caused by co-morbid disease. *Neurology* 2000; 54:S8–15.
Chesson AL, Jr., Ferber RA, Fry JM, et al. The indications for polysomnography and related procedures. *Sleep* 1997; 20:423-87.
Ferber R, Kryger M (Eds). *Principles and Practice of Sleep Medicine in the Child.* WB Saunders, 1995
Kryger MH, Roth T, Dement WC. (Eds). *Principles and Practice of Sleep Medicine.* WB Saunders, 2000.
Moldofsky H. Sleep and pain. *Sleep Med Rev* 2001; 5:387–98.
Malhotra A, Fogel RB, Pillar G, Winkelman JW. *Non Respiratory Disorders of Sleep. Pulmonary and Critical Care Update.* American College of Chest Physicians; Volume 14: Lesson 4, 1999.
Ohayon MM, Vecchierini MF. Daytime sleepiness and cognitive impairment in the elderly population. *Arch Intern Med* 2002 28;162:201–8.
Reynolds CF 3rd. Sleep and affective disorders. A mini review. *Psychiatr Clin North Am* 1987; 10:583–91.
Turek FW, Dugovic C, Zee PC. Current understanding of the circadian clock and the clinical implications for neurological disorders. *Arch Neurol* 2001; 58:1781–7.
Van Reeth O, Weibel L, Spiegel K, Leproult R, Dugovic C, Maccari S. Interactions between stress and sleep: from basic research to clinical situations. *Sleep Med Rev* 2000; 4: 201–19.
Vgontzas AN, Kales A. Sleep and its disorders. *Annu Rev Med* 1999; 50:387–400.

Sleep apnoea

American Academy of Sleep Medicine Task Force. Sleep-related breathing disorders in adults: recommendations for syndrome definition and measurement techniques in clinical research. The Report of an American Academy of Sleep Medicine Task Force. *Sleep* 1999; 22:667–89.

Barvaux VA, Aubert G, Rodenstein DO. Weight loss as a treatment for obstructive sleep apnoea. *Sleep Med Rev* 2000; 4: 435–52.

Bradley TD, Floras JS. Pathophysiologic and therapeutic implications of sleep apnea in congestive heart failure. *J Cardiac Failure* 1996; 2:223–40.

Chervin RD, Guilleminault C. Obstructive sleep apnea and related disorders. *Neurologic Clinics* 1996; 14:583–609.

Exar EN, Collop NA. The upper airway resistance syndrome. *Chest* 1999;115: 1127–39.

Fogel RB, White DP. Obstructive sleep apnea. *Adv Intern Med* 2000; 45:351–89.

Guilleminault C, Pelayo R. Sleep-disordered breathing in children. *Ann Med* 1998;30:350–6.

Kramer NR, Cook TE, Carlisle CC, Corwin RW, Millman RP. The role of the primary care physician in recognizing obstructive sleep apnea. *Arch Intern Med* 1999;159:965–8.

Lavie P. *The Breath of Life.* Yale University Press, New Haven, London, 2002.

Lavie P, Silverberg D, Oksenberg A, Hoffstein V. Obstructive sleep apnea and hypertension: from correlative to causative relationship. *J Clin Hypertens* 2001; 3:296–301.

Lavie P, Herer P, Hoffstein V. Obstructive sleep apnoea syndrome as a risk factor for hypertension: population study. *BMJ* 2000; 320:479–82.

Leung RS, Bradley TD. Sleep apnea and cardiovascular disease. *Am J Respir Crit Care Med* 2001 164:2147–65.

Martin TJ, Sanders MH. Chronic alveolar hypoventilation: a review for the clinician. *Sleep* 1995; 18:617–34.

Marcus CL. Sleep-disordered breathing in children. *Am J Respir Crit Care Med* 2001;164:16–30.

Messner AH, Pelayo R. Pediatric sleep-related breathing disorders. *Am J Otolaryngol* 2000; 21:98–107.

Malhotra A, Ayas NT, Epstein LJ. The art and science of continuous positive airway pressure therapy in obstructive sleep apnea. *Curr Opin Pulm Med* 2000; 6: 490–5.

Millman RP, Rosenberg CL, Kramer NR. Oral appliances in the treatment of snoring and sleep apnea. *Clin Chest Med* 1998;19:69–75.

Naughton MT, Bradley TD. Sleep apnea in congestive heart failure. *Clin Chest Med* 1998; 19:99–113.

Piper AJ, Stewart DA. An overview of nasal CPAP therapy in the management of obstructive sleep apnea. *Ear Nose Throat J* 1999; 78:776–8, 781–2, 784–90.

Redline S, Tishler PV. The genetics of sleep apnea. *Sleep Med Rev* 2000; 4: 583–602.

Sher AE. Surgical management of obstructive sleep apnea. *Prog Cardiovasc Dis* 1999; 41:387–96.

Troell RJ, Riley RW, Powell NB, Li K. Long-term results of surgical management of sleep disordered breathing: are our patients really benefiting? *Otolaryngol Clin North Am* 1998; 31: 1031–5.

Young T, Palta M, Dempsey J, Skatrud J, Weber S, Badr S. The occurrence of sleep-disordered breathing among middle-aged adults. *N Engl J Med* 1993;328: 1230–5.

Hypersomnia, general

Billiard M, Dauvilliers Y. Idiopathic hypersomnia. *Sleep Med Rev* 2001; 5:351–60.

Douglas NJ. 'Why am I sleepy?': sorting the somnolent. *Am J Respir Crit Care Med* 2001;163:1310–3.

El-Ad B, Korczyn AD. Disorders of excessive daytime sleepiness – an update. *J Neurol Sci* 1998;153:192–202.

Gadoth N, Kesler A, Vainstein G, Peled R, Lavie P. Clinical and polysomnographic characteristics of 34 patients with Kleine-Levin syndrome. *J Sleep Res* 2001;10:337–41.

Guilleminault C, Brooks SN. Excessive daytime sleepiness: a challenge for the practising neurologist. *Brain* 2001;124:1482–91.

Mahowald MW. What is causing excessive daytime sleepiness? Evaluation to distinguish sleep deprivation from sleep disorders. *Postgrad Med* 2000; 107: 108–10,115–8, 123.

Roth T, Roehrs TA. Etiologies and sequelae of excessive daytime sleepiness. *Clin Therapeutics* 1996; 18:562–76.

Narcolepsy

Choo KL, Guilleminault C. Narcolepsy and idiopathic hypersomnolence. *Clin Chest Med* 1998; 19:169–81.

Dement WC. The history of narcolepsy and other sleep disorders. *J Hist Neurosci* 1993;2:121–34.

Littner M, Johnson SF, McCall WV, et al. Practice parameters for the treatment of narcolepsy: an update for 2000. *Sleep* 2001;24:451–66.

Lin L, Hungs M, Mignot E. Narcolepsy and the HLA region. *J Neuroimmunol* 2001;117:9–20.

Mignot E. Genetic and familial aspects of narcolepsy. *Neurology* 1998; 50:S16–22.

Nishino S, Ripley B, Overeem S, Lammers GJ, Mignot E. Hypocretin (orexin) deficiency in human narcolepsy. *Lancet* 2000; 355:39–40.

Overeem S, Mignot E, Gert van Dijk J, Lammers GJ. Narcolepsy: clinical features, new pathophysiologic insights, and future perspectives. *J Clin Neurophysiol* 2001;18:78–105.

Thannickal TC, Moore RY, Nienhuis R, et al. Reduced number of hypocretin neurons in human narcolepsy. *Neuron* 2000; 27:469–74.

Periodic leg movements

Hening W, Allen R, Earley C, Kushida C, Picchietti D, Silber M. The treatment of restless legs syndrome and periodic limb movement disorder. An American Academy of Sleep Medicine Review. *Sleep* 1999; 22:970–99.

Provini F, Vetrugno R, Meletti S, et al. Motor pattern of periodic limb movements during sleep. *Neurology* 2001;57:300–4.

Trenkwalder C, Walters AS, Hening W. Periodic limb movements and restless legs syndrome. *Neurol Clin* 1996; 14:629–50.

Insomnia

Allen RP, Earley CJ. Restless legs syndrome: a review of clinical and pathophysiologic features. *J Clin Neurophysiol* 2001;18:128–47.

Bootzin RR, Perlis ML. Nonpharmacologic treatments of insomnia. *J Clin Psychiatry* 1992; 53:S37–41.

Chase JE, Gidal BE. Melatonin: therapeutic use in sleep disorders. *Ann Pharmacother* 1997; 31:1218–26.

Chesson A Jr, Hartse K, Anderson WM, et al. Practice parameters for the evaluation of chronic insomnia. An American Academy of Sleep Medicine (AASM) report. Standards of Practice Committee of the AASM. *Sleep* 2000 23:237–41.

Dement WC. The proper use of sleeping pills in the primary care setting. *J Clin Psychiatry* 1992; 53:S50–60.

Edinger JD, Wohlgemuth WK, Radtke RA, Marsh GR, Quillian RE. Cognitive behavioral therapy for treatment of chronic primary insomnia: a randomized controlled trial. *JAMA* 2001; 285:1856–64.

Gillin JC, Spinweber CL, Johnson LC. Rebound insomnia: a critical review. *J Clin Psychopharmacol* 1989; 9:161–72.

Hauri PJ. Insomnia. *Clin Chest Med* 1998; 19:157-68.

Hauri P (ed.) *Case Studies in Insomnia*. Kluwer Academic Plenum Publishers, 1991.

Lavie P. Sleep disturbances in the wake of traumatic events. *N Engl J Med* 2001;345:1825–32.

Kupfer DJ, Reynolds CF. Current concepts: management of insomnia. *N Engl J Med* 1997; 336:341–6.

Lichstein KL, Morin CM. *Treatment of Late-Life Insomnia*. Sage Publications, Thousands Oaks CA, 2000.

Mendelson WB, Jain B. An assessment of short-acting hypnotics. *Drug Saf* 1995; 13:257–70.

Mitler MM. Nonselective and selective benzodiazepine receptor agonists—where are we today? *Sleep* 2000; 23:S39–47.

Morin CM. *Insomnia*. Guilford Press, NY, 1996.

Richardson GS, Roth T. Future directions in the management of insomnia. *J Clin Psychiatry* 2001; 62:S39–45.

Morin CM, Culbert JP, Schwartz SM. Nonpharmacological interventions for insomnia: a meta-analysis of treatment efficacy. *Am J Psychiatry* 1994; 151:1172–80.

Morin CM, Colecchi C, Stone J, Sood R, Brink D. Behavioral and pharmacological therapies for late-life insomnia: a randomized controlled trial. *JAMA* 1999; 281: 991–9.

Noble S, Langtry HD, Lamb HM. Zopiclone. An update of its pharmacology, clinical efficacy and tolerability in the treatment of insomnia. *Drugs* 1998; 55: 277–302.

Ramchandani P, Wiggs L, Webb V, Stores G. A systematic review of treatments for settling problems and night waking in young children. *BMJ* 2000; 320:209–13.

Regestein QR, Monk TH. Delayed sleep phase syndrome: a review of its clinical aspects. *Am J Psychiatry* 1995; 152:602–8.

Richardson GS, Roth T. Future directions in the management of insomnia. *J Clin Psychiatry* 2001; 62:S39-45.

Sateia MJ, Doghramji K, Hauri PJ, Morin CM. Evaluation of chronic insomnia. An American Academy of Sleep Medicine review. *Sleep* 2000;23:243–308.

Wagner J, Wagner ML. Non-benzodiazepines for the treatment of insomnia. *Sleep Med Rev* 2000; 4:551–81.

Wagner J, Wagner ML, Hening WA. Beyond benzodiazepines: alternative pharmacologic agents for the treatment of insomnia. *Ann Pharmacother* 1998; 32:680–91.

Ware JC, Walsh JK, Scharf,MB, Roehrs T, Roth T, Vogel GW. Minimal rebound insomnia after treatment with 10-mg zolpidem. *Clin Neuropharmacol* 1997; 20:116–25.

Parasomnia

Bressman SB, et al. Treatment of hyperkinetic movement disorders. *Neurol Clin* 1990; 8:51–75.

Dyken ME, Rodnitzky RL. Periodic, aperiodic, and rhythmic motor disorders of sleep. *Neurology* 1992; 42:68–74.

Hublin C, Kaprio J, Partinen M, Koskenvu M. Parasomnias: co-occurrence and genetics. *Psychiatr Genet* 2001;11:65–70.

Llorente MD, Currier MB, Norman SE, Mellman TA. Night terrors in adults: phenomenology and relationship to psychopathology. *J Clin Psychiatry* 1992; 53:392–4.

Mahowald MW, Schenck CH. NREM sleep parasomnias. *Neurol Clin* 1996; 14:675–96.

Mahowald MW, Ettinger MG. Things that go bump in the night – the parasomnias revisited. *J Clin Neurophysiology* 1990;7:119–143.

Ohayon MM, Li KK, Guilleminault C. Risk factors for sleep bruxism in the general population. *Chest* 2001; 119:53–61.

Schenck CH, Mahowald MW. Review of nocturnal sleep-related eating disorders. *Int J Eating Disorders* 1994; 15:343–56.

Schenck CH, Mahowald MW. REM sleep parasomnias. *Neurol Clin* 1996; 14:697–720.

Schenck CH, Mahowald MW. Parasomnias. Managing bizarre sleep-related behavior disorders. *Postgrad Med* 2000; 107:145–56.

Tobias NE. Management of nocturnal enuresis. *Nurs Clin North Am* 2000; 35:37–60.

Scientific journals

Sleep – The official publication of the American Academy of Sleep Medicine and the Sleep Research Society. Both basic research and clinical papers

Journal of Sleep Research – The official publication of the European Sleep Research Society. Both basic research and clinical papers.

Sleep Medicine Reviews – A journal dedicated to review articles written by leading reseachers.

Sleep Medicine – A journal dedicated to clinical publications in sleep medicine.

Index